Working in Partnership

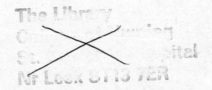

Working in Partnership

Clinicians and carers in the management
of longstanding mental illness

Liz Kuipers and Paul Bebbington

Heinemann Medical Books

For the patients, relatives and staff of Red Team

Heinemann Medical Books
An imprint of Heinemann Professional Publishing Ltd
Halley Court, Jordan Hill, Oxford OX2 8EJ

OXFORD   LONDON   SINGAPORE   NAIROBI
IBADAN   KINGSTON

First published 1990

British Library Cataloguing in Publication Data
Kuipers, Liz
Working in partnership: clinicians and carers in the
management of longstanding mental illness.
1. Mentally ill persons. Care
I. Title II. Bebbington, Paul
362.20425

ISBN 0 433 01606 X

Typeset by Best-set Typesetter Ltd, Hong Kong
Printed in Great Britain by Biddles Ltd, Guildford and
Kings Lynn

Contents

Preface

This book is intended to help psychiatric professionals who want to work with the relatives of those suffering from longstanding and severe mental illness like schizophrenia. It has a simple theme; that in the management of these conditions it is feasible and worthwhile to form alliances, not merely with patients, but with the relatives who live with them. These alliances should be therapeutic, operating for the benefit of the patient. They also mean that the professional is giving a service to the relatives.

Although the idea of partnership seems both reasonable and obvious, it has taken a long time to gain even a wary acceptance in the psychiatric professions.

A system of relationships is bound to be altered when a participant develops a severe mental disorder. Working with relatives in the way we propose carries an assumption about the effects of psychiatric illness within the family. The condition of sufferers will affect other family members, whose responses will in turn affect them. This seems self-evident to us as an extension of the ordinary social influence that human beings exert on one another.

These mutual influences have in any case been documented and quantified in research that now extends back for a generation. This research has two elements: the effect of mental illness on family members, and the influence of the family on the course and outcome of the disorder.

Professionals who concentrate on the behaviour and well-being of individual patients individually managed therefore only approach one side of the problem. They miss an opportunity for modifying the social environment in beneficial ways by enlisting the constructive aid of relatives. It is our view that we now know enough about how to do this for it to be a standard part of the long-term management of severe mental illness.

At the moment, relatively few psychiatric professionals do work with relatives as a routine part of this management. There appear to be two major barriers that prevent this happening. The first lies in the negative attitudes of professionals towards families. The second concerns their lack of skills in evaluating the problems of relatives and in helping with them.

One object of this book is thus to persuade readers that the families of their patients should be treated both as a therapeutic resource and as a legitimate focus of professional concern. The relevant literature makes this quite clear and is reviewed in the earlier part of the book.

The second, and larger part of this book sets out a range of strategies that can be used to define the problems relatives may face and to help develop ways of dealing with them. By providing this structure, we hope to encourage readers to involve relatives routinely in the management of patients with severe functional mental illness. The adaptation of ordinary professional interpersonal skills to achieve this takes time, but once the professional engages with relatives in a constructive way, a start has been made that can be built upon with practice.

Although we make reference to techniques of rehabilitation our account is not intended to be exhaustive. The book is meant rather to supplement standard texts (Wing and Morris, 1981; Lamb, 1982; Watts and Bennett, 1983; Shepherd, 1984; Hume and Pullen, 1986) and to bring rehabilitation into the context of patients' families.

Although much caring of the mentally ill is done by relatives, not all carers are blood relatives or spouses by any means: some of the most successful caring relationships are made by friends, landladies or home helps. People living in hostels are in a family of close relationships, both with the other residents and with staff. Staff members will themselves often form the most important social relationships for long-term patients. People with schizophrenic illnesses show a severe reduction in regular social contacts, down from a norm of perhaps 30 people to only 4 or 5 (Pattison et al., 1975; Beels, 1979; Henderson 1980). In this situation staff members might almost be defined as family, and indeed in our experience they often share the problems and difficulties of relatives. Anyone who is seen regularly and has some continued involvement with a patient, in terms of the commitment of time or the provision of care or help, therefore falls into our category of carer.

Being a carer implies considerable devotion of time and effort to patients. Along with this goes emotional investment and concomitant strong feelings of love, regard, concern, hatred, frustration, anger, guilt and sorrow. It is this combination of

emotional turmoil with the exhausting array of practical problems involved in living with the long-term mentally ill that renders
professional intervention both difficult and, in our opinion, necessary. A recent survey of carers of this group (MacCarthy et al.,
1990) found that practical help was often forthcoming (e.g.
housing, financial advice), but that emotional help was always
deficient. Whether this was because not enough was offered, or
because the need is too great to be satisfied is not known. It is
however very clear that the obvious requirement for long-term
help with these emotional needs has yet to be met by psychiatric
professionals.

The approach we advocate here is a pragmatic one, derived
from the research literature but illuminated by clinical experience. It draws on elements of behavioural skills training, on the
family approaches advocated by Haley (1976) and Minuchin
(1974), on the study of group processes and, probably most important, on common sense. It certainly does not offer guarantees,
but anyone working in this area will already know that an easy
success is hardly a realistic expectation: the approach aims at
giving a structure to professional interventions with families and
patients facing the very difficult and often unending task of coping
with long-term mental illness.

Within this framework, there can be no detailed rules. Therapists must become aware of the range of problems that beset
carers and their likely responses to them. This permits an intelli-
gent evaluation of the actual problems, responses and emotions
experienced by given relatives. On the basis of this information,
the actual process of intervening must be carried out flexibly.
Therapists must always be ready to change tack: to accept what
can be salvaged if their original approach looks like being unsuccessful, and to try another strategy in good time.

Our own approach to intervention with this group of relatives
relies essentially on three techniques. The first is cognitive re-
structuring — the use of information of various sorts to modify
the families' attitudes in a way that facilitates change by making
it possible for them to try new things. The second is the provision
of a safe forum in which relatives and carers can express their
feelings and emotional needs. This makes it possible to defuse
and contain emotions that operate to block beneficial changes in
their situation. The third technique is that of problem solving; in
some cases therapists may themselves suggest solutions to problems, but the ideal is to enhance the skills of families so that they

can themselves deal with difficulties as they arise. In practice, with relatives of patients with long-term illness, both therapists and carers contribute to the process of problem solving — the therapist is often part of the solution. These techniques of intervention are described in later chapters.

The first principle of intervention with the families of those with long-term mental illness is the obvious one of engagement — therapists cannot help families who refuse to see them. This can be a considerable problem with these families, who normally have a long history of experiences that make them justifiably suspicious of the clinician's intent. We deal with techniques of engagement at greater length in Chapter 4.

The second principle is for the therapist to accept that the time scale of intervention may have to be prolonged. The process of change is very likely to be slow. However, the adoption of a long time scale may mean that families' circumstances change incidentally, and the therapist must be alert to the possibility of using new situations to solve old problems.

Once the initial engagement has been achieved, focusing on some of the problems faced by patients' families is an effective way of understanding their situation, structure and dynamics. Subtle questioning may be needed to define the nature of particular problems, which will sometimes be presented in rather vague terms. Where more than one relative lives with a patient, they often see the problem in a very different light, and this demands clarification by the therapist.

After therapists have arrived at a reasonable idea of what the problem is, they must assess its place in the economy of the family. How does it handicap the patient and each member of the family? Who gains what from the continuation of the problem? Is it being reinforced in obvious or subtle ways? How does each member of the family feel about the problem? What would be gained if it were eliminated? If the problem were solved, would there be bad consequences for any member of the family? If it cannot be solved, are things likely to get worse and, if so, in what ways? It will very often be found that families have opted for solutions of least cost rather than of most benefit.

In general, once an idea of the range of problems faced by the family has been formed, the goals of treatment should be settled by a process of negotiation. Sometimes family members will be unrealistic, and the therapist may need to get them to change their expectations. This can sometimes be done by specifying intermediate goals. Families in any case often choose goals that are broad aspirations rather than specific targets. Therapists should build on this by formulating a series of intermediate or component steps that can be precisely specified. Aims couched in over-general terms do not lend themselves to the exact prescription of the sort of action that is feasible for the families to attempt.

Ultimately, a book like this can only provide guidelines about likely problems and feasible solutions, rather than a detailed prescription for action. We will have benefitted our readers if we can persuade them to relate what we write to their own clinical experiences, and in the process increase their flexibility of approach.

Liz Kuipers
Paul Bebbington

Part One

The Scientific Background

1·*Meeting Needs*

The decision to involve relatives in the management of those with persistent severe mental illness means that the needs of three groups of people must be considered: the patients, the relatives, and the staff. Each group will be exposed to considerable stress in one way or another, and this must be dealt with if engagement is to be effective. In this chapter, we consider the needs of each group. However, we concentrate on those of the relatives, as they are the most neglected. Knowing of the existence and nature of these needs is crucial to the establishment of the effective partnership between clinicians and carers that we advocate.

The Needs of Patients

The needs of patients with longstanding psychiatric illness have been dealt with at length by others (e.g. Wing, 1987). They suffer from multiple disadvantages. Before they can seriously be considered to belong to the long-term group, they must have had illness persisting for at least a year. However most will have been ill for many years. Although the prognosis of schizophrenia has probably improved during the last decades, only 25% will be in the best outcome group, and the remainder will have persistent disability or recurrent attacks (Wing, 1982). Nevertheless, five years after a first schizophrenic illness, 90% of sufferers are still living in the community and as many as two thirds will be with relatives (Kuipers and Bebbington, 1988). Likewise, a sizeable minority of people with severe affective disturbance go on to a chronic course (Bebbington, 1982; Lee and Murray, 1988; Kiloh et al., 1988; Mann and Cree, 1975).

The age range of these patients may be considerable. In our own service, we have patients as young as nineteen; most are somewhat older, and some have grown old in the service — we have one or two patients in their seventies. The problems they experience are likely to vary with age. The very young may have difficulties arising from 'frozen immaturity', whereas the elderly tend to have physical impairments as well as mental ones. They have all the ordinary problems of growing old on top of the difficulties in living in the community caused by mental illness.

Because these patients have been in contact with the services for a long time, many treatments will have been tried. At best they will have only been of limited success. There are many reasons for this — poor compliance with treatment, the resistance of particular consequences of the disorder to modification, and the existence of complicating secondary or incidental handicaps, such as physical disability, low educational level, a forensic history, alcohol abuse, low self esteem, or lack of confidence. In consequence, these patients experience a huge variety of problems, made more difficult to deal with as they rarely remain the same for long.

Up to 7% of patients may remain floridly psychotic, experiencing hallucinations and acting on delusions despite the use of every conceivable pharmacological treatment (Leff and Wing, 1971). The result may be scant or fleeting insight, turbulent or violent behaviour, persistent distress, a lack of cooperation leading to inconsistent medication or compulsory admission, and a lack of concentration that prevents the patient from engaging in constructive treatment.

The most common symptoms seen in this group are however the negative ones. These include anhedonia, reduced emotional responsiveness, social withdrawal, lack of energy and interest, poor concentration, and slow thinking. In the worst cases, they can lead to extreme self neglect, such that nutrition and health may be at considerable hazard. Negative and florid symptoms may coexist, either temporarily or permanently. However, there are no 'good' negative symptoms, and even at a moderate level they will impair restoration of function.

Over the years these patients are likely to be ascribed numerous diagnoses. In our experience, many have quite marked depressive and neurotic symptoms. These are often poorly recognized and poorly treated, and are in any case rather difficult to deal with. Anxiety may interact with delusions and indeed be attributed to delusional beliefs, making the usual treatments such as desensitization hard to apply.

In evaluating the progress of patients with persistent illnesses, it is useful to adopt the simple idea of 'staircases and landings' used by Wing (1987) to represent the stage reached by patients in relation to particular functions. The position of patients on the staircases varies according to the particular skill area under consideration. It is not to be assumed that because patients are good at one thing, they will be good at another. So, for example, one may have good self-care but poor occupational skills, another may be socially withdrawn but good at mechanical tasks. Many of our patients are rather good at certain leisure activities, such as placing bets, but poor at self-care. Care and intervention therefore has to be pitched at different levels in different areas. Moreover, the rate of progress in particular areas will also vary.

This emphasizes the need for the flexible and coordinated use of services to ensure that the patient will benefit.

Moreover, although we may hope for improvement, the maintenance of function and even the mere slowing of deterioration are equally valid objectives. There are many good and detailed descriptions of general rehabilitation practice (Royal College of Psychiatrists, 1980, 1987; Lamb, 1982; Watts and Bennett, 1983; Wing, 1987). In our group of patients, as well as the usual monitoring of the mental state and the effective provision of medication, attention must be directed at nutrition, physical health, self-care, practical skills, leisure, and accommodation. This may involve the provision of structured day care, drop-in facilities, and, in those cases who may be a danger to themselves or to others, secure containment. This group of patients poses particular problems of engagement: it is sometimes very difficult to keep them in contact with services. One need of these patients is therefore for effective outreach. This is especially important with current policies of community care that require greater survival skills and offer more opportunities for falling through the net.

The Needs of Carers

In large part, the needs of patients are met by carers. As a consequence, they themselves develop needs, and these are less often recognized, and certainly less often met. They have been clearly documented in a number of research studies evaluating the burden upon relatives brought about by living with someone who is mentally ill. This is usually referred to as 'burden' for short (Fadden et al., 1987a).

There is something odd about the literature on burden. Studies in this area date back over a third of a century, and we knew little less then than we do now. Nevertheless, a new study is completed every three years or so. It is as if we were constantly having to reinvent the wheel.

The reason for this probably lies in the fact that the findings of the studies, although remarkably consistent, are simply not taken on board by psychiatrists and their colleagues from related disciplines. They are certainly not incorporated into everyday clinical activities. In consequence, researchers, who in any case tend to be committed to the relatives' cause, feel the need to make the point ever more strongly. We can sympathize with this. There is certainly no doubt about the evidence that people are adversely affected by the experience of sharing their lives with a mentally ill relative, even though they may not complain much.

Severe mental illness almost always leads to the breakdown of the reciprocal arrangements that people maintain in their relationships. One person consequently ends up doing 'more than their fair share'. This may merely result in them taking on an overlarge proportion or number of shared tasks, but it usually also restricts their activities outside the relationship. Indeed, relatives are often affected in almost every area of their lives. As may be imagined, this change in pattern can be accompanied by a considerable sense of subjective dissatisfaction. However, there is considerable variation in the levels of distress (Platt, 1985).

What Relatives Have to Put up With

The degree of burden reported among the relatives of patients with persistent psychiatric disorders varies appreciably, but largely because different criteria are used for assessing its severity. However, the tenor of the literature leaves a consistent impression.

Mandelbrote and Folkard (1961a and 1961b) estimated the degree to which families were restricted or disturbed by the presence of schizophrenic patients in the home. Their assessment was fairly crude, but they reckoned over half their families could be rated as disturbed in some way, though only 2% of relatives reported severe stress.

Mills' (1962) study was of unselected psychiatric patients. Practically all were a source of anxiety to their relatives. More than half were described as 'difficult' at home, and only a small minority caused no practical difficulties. In Grad and Sainsbury's study (1963a,b), almost two thirds of the families had been experiencing hardship because the patient was living at home, and in one fifth the burden was severe.

Wing and his colleagues (1964b) followed the course of 113 schizophrenic patients for a year after discharge. Where patients returned to live with their families, social relations were strained in nearly two thirds of cases, often to the limit of what would ordinarily be regarded as tolerable.

Waters and Northover (1965) similarly reported that many of their schizophrenic men occasioned moderate to severe hardship to their relatives in terms of social embarrassment, inconvenience, and behaviour which frightened them or gave rise to tension in the family. Hoenig and Hamilton (1966, 1969) found that three quarters of their patients had some kind of adverse effect on the household.

The conclusion from these studies must therefore be that burden exists and is extensive. It is reflected in the high rates of divorce and separation in marriages where one patient is mentally ill. For example, in many cases observed by Brown and his colleagues (1966), the patient's illness had been instrumental in bringing about divorce or separation. The divorce and separation rates quoted in the study were three times the national average for female patients, four times for males.

However, in some ways, it is surprising that more marriages do not break up. In the study of Yarrow and his colleagues (1955a) several wives had contemplated separation or divorce, but all had decided to give the relationship another try. A similar adherence to the marriage, in the face of considerable difficulties and apparently meagre rewards, was noted by Fadden and her colleagues (1987b).

This degree of commitment to situations that cannot be very rewarding is remarkable, and should be borne in mind in the clinician's dealings with relatives and carers.

Effects on Social Relationships

One of the most damaging consequences of living with a relative with a persistent mental illness is the detriment to social and leisure activities. This was noted in the first study of the problem (Yarrow et al., 1955b): the wives of the patients in this study consistently believed that mental illness was stigmatized by others, and expressed fears of social discrimination. In consequence, a third of them adopted a pattern of 'aggressive concealment', making drastic changes in order to avoid or cut off former friends. Some even went so far as to move to a different part of town. Another third had told only members of the family, or close friends who either understood the problem or had been in a similar situation themselves.

A number of other studies have documented the restriction of social activity experienced by those who live with and care for patients with schizophrenia (e.g. Mandelbrote and Folkard, 1961a,b; Wing et al., 1964b; Waters and Northover, 1965) and this can be especially marked when the relative is an elderly parent (Leff et al., 1982). Similar findings have also been reported for spouses of a group of patients with persistent depressive disorders (Fadden et al., 1987b). These relatives spent over sixty hours a week in face-to-face contact with the patient, and were correspondingly socially isolated. Grad and Sainsbury (1963a,b) also found that the restrictions are not limited to those living with schizophrenic patients. The phenomenon of stigma probably contributes as much to this social isolation today as it did in 1955.

Financial Difficulties

These have been emphasized in a number of studies (Yarrow et al., 1955b; Mandelbrote and Folkard, 1961a,b; Mills, 1962; Hoenig and Hamilton, 1966, 1969; Stevens, 1972; Fadden et al., 1987b). To some extent, difficulties may arise because caring for a patient with a persistent psychiatric disorder limits opportunities for an adequate income. However, the most severe effects are seen when former breadwinners become ill, particularly if circumstances prevent the relative from taking over this role. The extent to which the families of psychiatric patients are financially impoverished ought not to be underestimated.

How do Relatives View the Illness?

In the nature of things, mental health professionals accept that behaviour can be symptomatic of illness. However, what we take for granted requires a major shift in attitude for relatives. Clausen and his colleagues (1955a) pointed to the difficulties the wives in their study experienced in understanding their husbands' actions. Their attitudes concerning the normality of such unfamiliar behaviour fluctuated continually, probably because of the overlap between the symptoms of mental illness and normal patterns of behaviour. At first, they tended to go for explanations in terms of physical difficulties, or character problems such as their husband being weak or lacking in will-power (Yarrow et al., 1955a). The authors note the psychological impact on the wife of having to consider her own possible role in the development of her husband's disorder, and of contemplating her future as the 'wife of a mental patient'.

The adjustment in attitudes that is required of relatives cannot be made easier by their own emotional turmoil. It is clear from the study described above that the wives experienced anxiety, guilt and feelings of rejection towards their husbands as a consequence of the illness. Most of the relatives described by Creer and Wing (1974) had also at various times experienced anger at the way their lives had been spoiled, and grief when they recalled what the patient had been like before the onset of illness. In the study of Fadden and her colleagues (1987b), many of the spouses of depressed patients expressed a sense of loss, as if they had been physically bereft of the person they had married. Anger and guilt were also prominent.

It is apparent from these accounts, and from others scattered throughout this literature, that the intrusion of mental illness into the family is a trauma that relatives have considerable difficulty (and little help) in adjusting to. Moreover, things may not become easier with the passage of time. Hoenig and Hamilton (1966, 1969) found that the likelihood of some objective burden increased the longer the patient remained ill. Mandelbrote and Folkard (1961a,b) similarly reported that more families came to be rated as disturbed as time passed during their four year follow-up period.

Burdensome Symptoms

Schizophrenia and other severe mental illnesses show a whole range of symptoms of different types. What are the sorts of symptoms that relatives find most wearing? There is fairly good agreement about this in the published studies, with burdensome symptoms falling in to two groups — publicly embarrassing symptoms and symptoms of withdrawal.

A common concern of the relatives in Mills' (1962) study was that patients might be a danger to themselves or others, and problems frequently arose with neighbours as a result of the patients' behaviour. Many relatives complained of disturbed nights, but reported that practical problems caused less difficulties than the patients' 'strange fancies' or 'dumb apathy'. Those patients who did not often speak created more distress than those who spoke too much, though the latter caused suffering too.

In Grad and Sainsbury's (1963a,b) study, patients with psychosis presented more of a problem than those with neurotic disorders. The symptoms found to be associated with a rating of severe burden were aggression, delusions, hallucinations, confusion and an incapacity for self-care. However, the problems families complained of most often were not the symptoms usually associated in the public mind with mental illness, such as violent or socially embarrassing behaviour, but rather the frustrating depressive and hypochondriacal preoccupations exhibited by patients. Brown and his colleagues (1966) found the number of problems and the distress experienced by relatives were closely related to the degree of disturbed behaviour shown by the schizophrenic patients in their study. Hoenig and Hamilton (1966, 1969) confirmed that relatives most frequently reported both aggressive behaviour and extreme seclusiveness of withdrawal as causing problems.

Creer and Wing (1974) found it was the 'negative' symptoms that caused most trouble for the relatives of their patients with schizophrenia — symptoms associated with social withdrawal, such as lack of conversation, underactivity, slowness and having few leisure interests. The other group of problem symptoms were socially embarrassing behaviours and the more obviously disturbed behaviours. The fact that relatives find 'negative' symptoms of schizophrenia very hard to cope with was again confirmed by Vaughn (1977), who did a content analysis of critical remarks made by relatives. Only one third of the remarks concerned delusions, hallucinations or other florid symptoms, whereas two thirds referred to behaviour such as lack of communication, affection, interest and initiative. Relatives were largely unable to view these deficiencies as part of the illness, but saw them rather as personality attributes which were under the patient's voluntary control. They disparaged the patients as 'lazy', 'selfish' and 'useless'.

In depressive illness, there are also symptoms which can in a broad sense be called negative, such as social withdrawal, quiet misery and so on. It is of interest that Fadden and her colleagues (1987b) reported that it was again symptoms of this type that relatives found most difficult to deal with, although florid and embarrassing behaviour was also hard to tolerate.

It can be seen that a consistent picture emerges from these accounts. Whereas relatives are apprehensive of florid symptoms, the suppressive effect of mental illness on behaviour also causes severe problems, and this is partly due to the difficulty which relatives have in attributing such effects to mental illness.

Do Relatives have the Support of the Mental Health Services?

In all this literature a link can be seen between the tolerance of relatives, and the lack of support given by the professionals caring for the patient. The lack of complaint often indicates pathetically low expectations of assistance.

The tolerance of relatives is observed again and again. Mills (1962) noted that relatives accepted their burdens in spite of the great sacrifices involved and, in protecting patients, endured really difficult behaviour. They sought re-admission only as a last resort. Wing and his colleagues (1964) emphasized that relatives did their best to put up with very disturbed behaviour, complained little and were willing to take on the role of nurse, frequently at the cost of considerable discomfort and distress.

Waters and Northover (1965) remarked on this tolerance of disturbed behaviour, and Hoenig and Hamilton (1966, 1969) similarly found that almost a quarter of the households carrying a good deal of objective burden made no complaint.

This certainly reflects the families' tolerance towards mentally ill members, but it also signifies something more sinister. Brown and his colleagues (1966) warn against assuming patients are better off at home just because the majority of relatives do not complain:

> The fact that there is this lack of complaint cannot be interpreted as a justification of community care.

Hoenig and Hamilton discovered that among those people who felt that nothing more could be done for them, three quarters suffered some objective burden, and almost a half complained of subjective burden. This shows the lack of expectation of help on the part of these relatives, and in fact only 7% of relatives in the study made any complaint about services.

Brown and his colleagues (1966) felt strongly that too much was sometimes being asked of relatives who, however, did not complain, either because they were too ashamed to talk about their problems or because they had concluded that no effective help would be offered. Relatives clearly needed expert aid, which they received only when their difficulties had reached a crisis.

Creer and Wing (1974) likewise reported that the reasons relatives of their schizophrenic patients rarely complained about their difficulties was not so much simple tolerance as shame, guilt, and the denial of problems. However, a disturbingly common reason for their acquiescent behaviour was their unfavourable experience of trying to obtain help. Virtually none of the relatives had received advice from professionals on the management of difficult behaviour, and those who worked out methods of dealing with problems did so by a painful process of trial and error. The authors concluded that there is no general recognition of the fact that relatives were functioning as 'primary care' agents, and suggested the introduction of a counselling scheme that would provide families with information and strategies for dealing with difficult situations.

A further study of long-term patients specifically examined how relatives felt about providing support — whether they were content, resigned or dissatisfied (Creer et al., 1982). These relatives too were coping with very difficult behaviours, for the most part without complaint. The authors were particularly concerned about the failure of professionals to meet relatives' needs, including those for practical assistance and advice, for emotional support, and for providing them with occasional breaks from their demanding task. They emphasized that no professional group was concerned with the problems of relatives in their own right, and that services were almost exclusively patient-oriented.

Wing (1982) reiterates the problems faced by relatives who have no training in dealing with difficult behaviour, who unlike hospital staff are 'on duty' all the time, and whose emotional involvement with the patient makes it difficult for them to remain neutral in their interactions with patients. Once again he advocates that professionals should make themselves aware of the real problems that arise in families.

A number of other authors have drawn clear inferences from their findings for the services that ought to be provided for the families of mental patients. Mandelbrote and Folkard (1961a,b) recommended that the burden on families should be lightened by arranging facilities to take the patient from the home for part of the day, and that more social workers were needed to deal with interpersonal problems within the families.

Mills (1962) was also of the opinion that relatives needed relief part of the day, at night, or during crises, and that these patients remained in the community only at the cost of considerable hardship. Her conclusion runs:

> If patients are more often to be treated from their own homes, then their families should not have to bear without help the severe practical problems and strains.

Waters and Northover (1965) regarded the lack of sustained support of patients' families as one of the important shortcomings of the community after-care provided for the patients. These papers were both written a quarter of a century ago, but there is no evidence that services have improved since then. The implications are stark.

The Behaviour of Professionals Towards Relatives

It is clear from what has gone before that professionals do not provide much help for relatives. The early American study quoted above (Clausen et al., 1955b) examined how this lack of provision was related to the communication between wives and their husbands' psychiatrists, and to the attitudes which each held towards the other (Deasy and Quinn, 1955). An analysis of the requests made by wives revealed that the majority were efforts to secure information regarding aetiology, diagnosis and prognosis, and advice on how to deal with the patient when he returned home. The remaining requests were either for help with personal problems or attempts to change the course of hospitalization. However, in almost two thirds of cases, the wives expressed dissatisfaction because they did not get the information they required or because the doctors were inaccessible. Most psychiatrists considered it reasonable that wives should expect information, and knew they did not always fulfill the needs of patients' families, either because of their heavy workload or because the nature of psychiatric illness made it difficult to answer many of the questions posed. Nevertheless the 23 psychiatrists interviewed gave their attention almost exclusively to their patients, and contacted relatives only in the early stages of hospitalization to secure information. Although they agreed that wives needed help from some source, they did not see this as their responsibility. When asked to describe the characteristics of a 'good' wife, they used terms such as 'she has insight into her husband's condition, lets the doctors alone, cooperates with the hospital's plans for the patient'. A 'bad' wife on the other hand was someone who 'exhibits signs of emotional distress, tries to thwart the hospital, takes up a great deal of the doctor's time'. These statements seem to miss the point somewhat. Deasy and Quinn (1955) reported that the psychiatrists frequently felt they had to protect patients from their wives, as they believed that factors in the relationship had contributed to the illness.

It can be imagined that these attitudes, whatever their level of justification, do not lead to the meeting of relatives' needs. Although no subsequent study has looked specifically at professional attitudes, these themes continue to arise in reports of relatives dealings with staff.

Community Care and the Burdens of Relatives

The impetus for many of the studies described here was provided by the move towards community care. It is obvious that if more patients are in the community, more relatives will be in the position of having to care for them and will experience burden in consequence. A worrying finding, however, emerges from the first study specifically designed to examine the differential effects of a community-oriented service and a more traditional hospital-based service on the relatives of psychiatric patients (Grad and Sainsbury, 1963a,b). Not only were more people caring for relatives in the first scheme, but their degree of burden was actually greater. The authors reckoned that this was because the burden on families in the traditional hospital approach was lightened by regular home visits by social work staff, while this was not the case in the community-based service.

The Mental Health of Relatives

While not all relatives behave in the same way, it is the nature of the burden placed on them that leads some to resort to ineffective strategies of coping. There are direct consequences for the relatives' own mental health. This has been documented particularly for those married to depressed or neurotic partners (Kreitman, 1964; Kreitman et al., 1970; Ovenstone, 1973a; Fadden et al., 1987b), but has also been noted for those living with schizophrenic patients (Brown et al., 1966; Hoenig and Hamilton, 1966, 1969; Stevens, 1972; Creer and Wing, 1974).

The Burden of Depressive Symptoms

The outome of affective illness is less good than commonly believed (Bebbington, 1982; Lee and Murray, 1988; Kiloh et al., 1988). In consequence, a fair proportion of longstay patients have predominantly affective conditions (Mann and Cree, 1975). Moreover, in our experience, many patients with longstanding illnesses that have been given other diagnoses do experience major symptoms of anxiety and depression.

There is little information about the specific effects of depression on the family of the patient (Kuipers, 1986). The literature deals exclusively with the effects on spouses, although this may not be inappropriate, as depressive patients are much more likely to be married and living with the marital partner than are people with schizophrenia. In these marriages there is frequently conflict (Hinchcliffe et al., 1978), particularly, over role functions (Ovenstone, 1973b) and a high level of dependence (Birtchnell and Kennard, 1983). With increasing pathology on the part of the husband fewer joint decisions are made (Collins et al., 1971), and the wives of depressive patients have significantly less independent social activity than controls (Nelson et al., 1970).

Fadden and her colleagues (1987b) have recently conducted a pilot study of the spouses of persistently depressed patients of specified types. Their findings show striking parallels with the findings on schizophrenia, and emphasize the severity of the burden borne by spouses and the noticeably adverse effect upon their mental health shown in a high prevalence of depressive and anxiety states.

Towards Helping Relatives

Although a lot is now known about relatives' difficulties, less has been written about the best strategies for relatives to use in dealing with their probems and of how, even if professionals knew what to advise, they could ensure their advice was adopted.

In their review of research on burden, Kreisman and Joy (1974) speak of the 'scatter-shot' approach on the part of researchers who have failed to follow through on promising leads in their own data:

> This lack of sustained interest has left us with fundamental pieces of information missing.

The results of this ignorance have been considerable — for relatives and for patients.

A number of main points can be summarized from the literature on the effects of psychiatric illness upon families living with mental patients. There was actually a more widespread interest in the topic in the late 1950's and early 1960's when community care programmes were first introduced. Schizophrenic patients constitute the only group in which interest in family burden has been sustained, although there is evidence that families of other patient groups are also affected to a major extent by the patient's illness (e.g. Orford, 1986).

It is clear that families typically put up with a great deal of difficult behaviour and that they frequently find the less clearcut symptoms very hard to tolerate. They often lack knowledge about the nature of the patient's illness, but get little help from professionals in the management of difficult behaviour except in times of crisis. In spite of all this they rarely make complaints. Coping with their relative's problems frequently results in adverse effects on their own health, both physical and psychological. From the first studies to the most recent, the point has been made repeatedly that relatives must not be asked to bear these burdens unassisted, and that they should be provided with more help from professionals. A prerequisite of helping in this way is a knowledge of the problems that are in fact faced by relatives, and there are plenty of pointers from the studies on burden. More guidance can be secured from investigations of the effect that relatives have on the patients they live with, as we shall show in succeeding chapters.

What then are the sorts of services that relatives should be able to expect? First, like the patient, they may require outreach. They may be quite suspicious of the intentions of staff, usually because of previous bad experiences. Much of this book is devoted to this problem of engagement.

Once engaged, they may have a range of practical needs. So,

help with accommodation may dictate liaison with social services, housing associations, or housing departments. Debt may require the services of a debt counsellor provided by the Citizen's Advice Bureau. The latter may be called in to advise also on benefits. These days benefits are a particular nightmare, with complex rules of entitlement and little enough available even after a successful assessment. Problems over childcare may require practical assistance from a variety of sources and liaison with the Health Visitor.

In general the psychiatric services are quite good at meeting practical needs of this sort (McCarthy et al., 1990). However, nothing that has been mentioned so far has much to do with severe mental illness. Ironically, the psychiatric services are most likely to fall down precisely in meeting those needs of relatives that arise from the patients' mental condition. Many carers want to be involved alongside the professional team in the care of their relatives. They need to feel that they can liaise with staff aware of the patients' problems and willing to take the carers' difficulties and potential contributions seriously. They want to be involved in decisions about treatment, to be contributors rather than the passive recipients of such decisions. The staff team must have a degree of continuity so that the relative does not have to keep going over the same old material. This implies a commitment on the part of the team to long-term contact. Good patient care and good liaison with the relative will often prevent crises, but carers need to feel that they have ready access to an emergency service if things do go wrong. They should certainly not feel themselves in a position where their only option is to call the police. Particularly as they grow older or fragile, carers may need the relief and the rest afforded by respite admission.

Sometimes relatives may have had more than they can take. It should not be assumed that they inevitably want to remain involved, and if they do not, this decision has to be respected. They may not wish to have the patient home again to live with them: under these circumstances it is up to staff to discover and support the extent to which the relatives now wish to be involved. This must be done with sensitivity, as in such cases relatives may misinterpret the invitation to attend a ward review as an ultimatum about taking the patient back. Such situations are surprisingly rare: most carers carry on gladly in the face of considerable burdens.

The Needs of Staff

Working with the long-term mentally ill can be extremely wearing for staff members, and a good multidisciplinary team takes account of this. The stresses must not be underestimated. The job involves dealing with people whose problems can appear insuperable and without limit. Patients may be very demanding, while showing low levels of cooperation and gratitude. The staff's personal safety may sometimes be in jeopardy. Some patients will deteriorate, but they must still be looked after. Others may improve and go to other placements, only to return worse than ever. The team is then left to pick up the pieces after the failures of their professional counterparts elsewhere. With particular patients staff may have to go back to square one, time after time. Some sufferers sabotage attempts to help them, leaving staff having to cope with rejection. Even where treatment is successful, change may be slow and difficult to see.

There are many parallels between the situation of staff as we have described it and that of the caring relatives. The attention of the staff, however, is split between several patients, and they therefore have the possibility of progress on some fronts even if denied it elsewhere. In any case, staff like relatives must guard against burnout — the onset of pessimism, loss of interest, enthusiasm and purpose, a sense of having become bogged down, and the feeling that they have lost competence and all capacity for fresh ideas (Lamb, 1982; Perlman and Hartman, 1982; Jackson et al., 1986). This problem is often compounded because the staff members in closest contact with patients are the most junior, who are constantly having to deal with difficult situations, perhaps at the margins of their competence.

The net result of this may be frequent absenteeism and high staff turnover, with consequent ill effects on the morale of the team as a whole. Such situations drastically reduce the capacity of the team to deliver the goods. It is not feasible to provide a service involving relatives after the fashion described in this book unless the team is functioning well. The structure and operations of the team must be planned to minimize the possibility of burn-out and low morale.

Guidelines for this have been set out elsewhere (Watts and Bennett, 1983). Dealing with the problems of long-term mental illness virtually demands a team set-up, and a democratic one at that. The ideal management structure is Japanese, whereby individuals are acknowledged to possess specific skills, but the distinction between professional groups is deliberately blurred. Members of different disciplines share out tasks that do not require special expertise, whether they are boring and routine, or interesting and innovative.

It is a crucial function of an effective team to prevent the isolation of its members. Decisions about issues of patient management are finalized on a team basis, so that the responsibility is shared even where the decision is implemented by a single member of staff. Problems will always arise, and a multidisciplinary team that deals badly with failure puts its members at risk. The organization of therapeutic endeavour on a team basis is potentially a great strength, although sometimes not used properly. Ideally it should mean that responsibilities are shared and no-one is working in isolation. It is perilous in dealing with the long-term group of patients to allow the burden to be borne silently by individual workers. Staff must feel free to share the difficulties, and this in turn is dependent on the culture provided by the team. It should not be seen as an appropriate machismo for individual staff members to have to cope with everything on their own. Staff should feel able to say they are not coping, without fear of criticism and in the expectation of support. No-one can cope with everything.

Team support can be made readily available through the provision of a proper structure. There should be a forum, perhaps weekly, devoted specifically to the discussion of problems and the sharing of burdens, and a culture should be fostered in which members of staff feel it is safe to reveal their worries.

There should also be clear procedures for dealing with disasters like being hit or intimidated. Staff should feel that it is all right to be upset by an unpleasant incident, and dealing with upset should not be regarded as an out-of-hours activity, but part of the mainstream of the team's function.

Most teams have some degree of staff turnover built in, and this is probably right: new people are needed in the system as a source of fresh ideas, and the danger of staff becoming institutionalized should be avoided. The team format makes staff turnover easier to deal with. Nevertheless, a continuity of philosophy if not of personnel is essential to efficient functioning. Working with the long-term group is not about doing novel things, but about doing the same thing over and over to ensure the desired outome.

This type of organization emphasizes the role of partnership within the team. This should be a reflection of a wider partnership of staff, carers, and patients. There is naturally some overlap of the functions of each within the partnership, and this overlap should be maximized. Staff and carers should end up doing rather similar things, albeit in different locations. This certainly does not mean that staff abrogate responsibility. They must remain in control, though not controlling, as this is necessary to the sense of safety of carers and patients.

Offering a service that includes rather than excludes relatives requires decisions about what will be acceptable to all concerned. This will be different for different families, but the principles remain the same. In our view, all interventions should be planned in the light of this idea of partnership.

2· The Influence of Relatives on the Patient's Wellbeing

In this chapter we will review investigations of social influence in general, and influence of the family in particular, on the course of the patient's illness. These studies have given us a considerable knowledge of the circumstances that may provoke relapse.

Social Influences on the Course of Severe Psychiatric Disorder

In the 1950's, a number of theories were put forward linking social factors with the onset of schizophrenia. They were all marked by a considerable ambitiousness. They tried to provide a virtually complete explanation of the emergence of the disease. Early experience was held to result in ways of seeing (and consequently of interacting with) the social world that correspond to the observed symptoms of schizophrenia.

Bateson and his colleagues (1956) proposed that schizophrenia was the result of the family's 'double bind' communication. Wynne and Singer (1963, 1965) also focused on communication difficulties and found that parents of people with schizophrenia had a 'fragmented' or 'amorphous' style of communication. Lidz (1957) claimed that such parents showed both 'schism' and 'skew' in their marriages, together with a narcissistic egocentricity. Finally, Laing and Esterson (1964) considered schizophrenia to be an understandable response to particular pressures in the family and in society at large.

For good reasons, these theories have now become unfashionable. Hirsch and Leff (1975) extensively reviewed the experimental evidence for them, and concluded that the oddities of the parents were not marked, and almost certainly not the cause of the condition. They thought there was reasonable support for a few rather modest relationships, including an increase in conflict and disharmony between the parents of schizophrenic patients, and in concern and protectiveness in their mothers, both in their current situation and before they fell ill.

These seem likely to be mere reactions to abnormalities in their offspring, which may have predated the development of obvious schizophrenia, but nevertheless formed part of the same process.

Finally, although the work of Wynne and Singer (1963, 1965) strongly suggested that parents of schizophrenic patients communicate abnormally, Hirsch and Leff (1975) were themselves unable to replicate their most definite findings. This has been the only independent attempt to test out these 'grand' social theories of the origins of schizophrenia.

A major problem of these early investigations is that causal direction is impossible to establish from retrospective studies. Other workers have attempted to get round this by using prospective studies. However, these are expensive, as most of the people laboriously followed up will never develop schizophrenia. A less costly approach involves following up families with children who may be at 'high risk' of developing schizophrenia (e.g. Venables, 1977; Goldstein, 1985). These, however, have their own problems, such as the length of time required to complete the study, high drop out rates, and the ethics of not intervening (Shakow, 1973).

One such study has actually been reported by Doane and her colleagues (1981 — see also Goldstein, 1987). They followed up adolescents thought to be at increased risk of developing schizophrenia, namely, those attending a psychiatric out-patient department for disturbed behaviour. They have now reported results available after a fifteen year interval. Only four adolescents developed definite schizophrenia in this time, but parental abnormalities of communication and affective style, and an approximate measure of Expressed Emotion (see below), all rated at induction, were clearly associated with the later emergence of schizophrenic spectrum disorders.

However, it is not clear what these findings actually say about the causes of schizophrenia, particularly if a narrower and more usual definition is used. It is possible that the more disturbed adolescents drew extreme reactions from their parents, and incidentally were also those who went on to develop the disease.

These studies are now to be seen as interesting failures. In many ways, they were laudable: they did at least have the effect of obtaining acceptance for a social dimension to the disorder, opening the door for more refined hypotheses.

However, they also seem to have been responsible for a very unfortunate sea change in the attitudes of professionals towards families. They provided explanations couched in terms which could be (and were) interpreted as a moral reproach. Concepts like the double bind, communication deviance, and the 'schizophrenogenic' mother were not elaborated with enough care to avoid the imputation of censure. This is particularly evident in popular representations of these ideas, for instance, in Ken Russell's film 'Family Life'.

We suspect that clinicians have read this literature in a cursory way, perhaps even at second hand. This leaves little but the idea that relatives are in some way to blame for their patients' condition. Thus in the 1959 edition of an influential texbook, Arieti felt able to state that the majority of cases of schizophrenia were the result of the mothers' behaviour towards their offspring.

To believe that relatives by their behaviour actually 'cause' schizophrenia is no longer feasible. Apart from any other consideration, the evidence for major genetic and physical environmental components is now well-founded. Nevertheless, this change is really one of relative emphasis: current theories certainly hold that social influences act on the manifestation of disorder, and that the behaviour of relatives has a role in this. We must therefore return to the issue of blameworthiness later, when we have described the more modern theories.

Social Influences on the Timing and Course of Schizophrenia

Social theories of schizophrenia with more modest aims have had a larger success. They start from the sensible position that social influences act together with factors at other levels to determine at least the timing, and possibly the fact, of schizophrenic breakdown. They rely on the concept of psychosocial stress, in particular as it is measured in terms of 'life events' and 'Expressed Emotion'. They thus reflect the widely held clinical opinion that people with schizophrenia are, despite the social withdrawal seen in many cases, very responsive to their social environment.

Life Events

There are sources of evidence other than direct studies of life events to suggest that changes in the social environment may lead to the emergence of schizophrenic symptoms in susceptible individuals. One of the most interesting is that acute florid symptoms may reappear in patients subjected to too much pressure in rehabilitation programmes, or discharged before they are ready (Wing et al., 1964a; Stevens, 1973; Goldberg et al., 1977). We have reviewed the role of psychosocial events in schizophrenia in detail elsewhere (Bebbington and Kuipers, 1988). The evidence is not as good as it might be, but on balance specific life event studies do support the belief that stress has some part in precipitating episodes of schizophrenia. Some studies show a positive association between antecedent life events and onset, others do not, and it is difficult to reconcile these results because the studies are all flawed in one way or another. The work of Brown and Birley (1968) although conducted many years ago has never really been bettered. They used fairly sophisticated methods for the day, and reported an increase in events, limited to the 3-week period before onset. This finding has largely been corroborated by the enormous WHO collaborative study (Bebbington, 1987; Day et al., 1987). The remaining studies attempting to link events to onset can be readily summarized in tabular form (Table 2.1). It is plain that a definitive study of life events in schizophrenia has yet to appear.

Brown and his colleagues (Brown et al., 1973, Brown and Harris, 1978) believe that life events have a 'triggering' effect in schizophrenia, whereas they might well be formative in depression. By this they mean that dispositional factors play the larger part in schizophrenia, and life events merely aggravate a strong pre-existing tendency. As triggers, events are seen as precipitating something that would have occurred before long for other reasons: they simply bring onset forward by a short period, and perhaps make it more abrupt. This makes considerable sense in the light of clinical experience: schizophrenic symptoms do indeed seem to recur if sufferers have to adapt to disruptions in their lives.

The idea that stress influences the course of schizophrenia does in our opinion receive rather better, indeed impressive, support from the literature on Expressed Emotion. This is a measure of family interaction, and is thus very relevant to the approach to the management of long-term illness proposed in this book.

Table 2.1 Life event studies in schizophrenia

Author	Location	N. of subjects	Case selection	Definition of onset	Life event measure	Period of analysis	Control group
Brown and Birley 1968	S London	50	Kraepelinian criteria based on PSE. First admissions and re-admissions	Normal-psychotic neurotic-psychotic or minor psychotic Onset within 3 months of admission, datable to within 1 week	Semistructured interview (early version of LEDS — Brown and Harris 1978)	3 months prior to onset in 3 week subdivisions	325 selected from local firms (ie imperfectly random)
Jacobs and Myers 1976	New Haven	62	Schizophrenia 'broadly defined': first admissions	Onset dated to within days based on emergence or exacerbation of symptoms and changes in social functioning	Modified version of Holmes & Rahe (1967) inventory given at interview	1 year prior to onset in 6 month subdivisions	62 matched for age, sex, social class, ethnicity, from random population sample
Malzacher et al. 1981	Zurich	33	Clinical definition, cf Brown & Birley 1968: first admissions	Emergence of psychotic symptoms	Life event inventory based on Tennant & Andrews (1976)	6 months prior to onset in 3 month subdivisions	33 matched for age, sex, marital status from random population sample
Canton and Fraccon 1985	Venice	54	DSMIII criteria: not all first admissions	Not defined	Life event inventory based on Paykel (1971) given at interview	6 months before admission or interview	54 normal normotensive subjects from hypertensive screening clinic matched for age, sex, social class marital status

Table 2.1 (con't)

Author	Location	N. of subjects	Case selection	Definition of onset	Life event measure	Period of analysis	Control group
Al Khani et al. 1986	Riyadh	48	Narrow operational definition: 92% CATEGO S+: not all first admissions	Exactly as Brown & Birley (1968)	WHO life events schedule given at interview	6 months prior to onset in 3 month sub-divisions; 3 months in 3 week sub-divisions	62 members of local community: imperfectly random sample
Chung et al. 1986	Sydney	15	DSMIII criteria: not all first admissions	Onset within 12 months: 'accurately' datable. normal-psychotic, normal-prodromal minor-major psychotic	LEDS (Brown & Harris 1978)	6 months, 13 weeks, 4 weeks prior to onset	Matched for age, sex, partly from local population, partly surgical patients
Day et al. 1987	Multicentre	386 from 9 centres	Broad range of psychotic cases, classified by local clinical diagnosis and CATEGO. Discrepant classifications in up to 28% of cases	Onset within 6 months, datable to within 1 week. normal-psychotic minor neurotic-psychotic; minor psychotic-major psychotic	WHO life events schedule given at interview	3 months prior to onset in 3 week sub-divisions	No controls

Expressed Emotion

The ideas behind our current concept of Expressed Emotion (EE) are now quite old, and have been reviewed at length elsewhere (Kuipers, 1979; Hooley, 1985; Leff and Vaughn, 1985; Koenigsberg and Handley, 1986; Kuipers and Bebbington, 1988; Vaughn, 1989). The story is an interesting one. It started with an unexpected finding, which was then seized upon, leading first to a series of increasingly sophisticated corroborative studies, finally to planned interventions with families (and to this book).

The original finding was reported in a study by Brown and his colleagues (Brown, 1959; Brown et al., 1958) of the prognosis of male mental patients with a variety of discharge arrangements. They found however, against expectation, that patients who went back to live with parents or spouses did surprisingly badly; they also noticed that this effect seemed to depend on the amount of contact between relative and patient — in other words, it was apparently dose-related. They therefore tentatively concluded that certain intense relationships might increase the risk of relapse.

Brown and his colleagues (1962) subsequently developed a semi-structured interview to assess the emotional atmosphere in the home. They thought that from this they would be able to identify specific qualities of the relationship that might be important in relation to relapse. The interview was refined and validated, and became the Camberwell Family Interview (CFI — Brown and Rutter, 1966; Rutter and Brown, 1966). Ratings were made of relatives according to the number of Critical Comments and of Positive Remarks they made, their overall Warmth, Hostility, and Emotional Overinvolvement, and the degree of Dissatisfaction they expressed in the interview. A composite rating of Expressed Emotion was derived from the ratings of Critical Comments, Hostility and Emotional Overinvolvement. Using this, Brown and his colleagues (1972) were able to predict relapse rates in a follow-up study of schizophrenic patients returning to their homes. Fifty eight per cent of patients returning to high EE homes relapsed, compared to 16% of those living with low EE relatives. The dose effect was found again: face to face contact of more than 35 hours per week increased the relapse rate in those patients living with high EE relatives.

This result was impressive: could it be due to initial differences in the patients that in time brought out different responses from the relatives? The authors did consider this, but found that the difference in outcome persisted after controlling for the patients' previous work impairment and behavioural disturbance.

The findings were almost exactly replicated by Vaughn and Leff (1976a) in a smaller study comparing a group of depressed neurotics with schizophrenic patients. As they used the same methods as the 1972 study, they were able to combine the data to give a larger sample (128). This allowed them to explore whether medication might modify relapse rates through providing protection against the effects of the family environment.

These results are shown in Figure 2.1. The implications are: first, relapse in schizophrenia may indeed be modified by social circumstances; secondly, patients with a high risk of relapse could be identified; and thirdly, since factors associated with relapse had been pinpointed, so also had the targets of a possible intervention programme. These targets comprise the effective provision of medication, a reduction of face-to-face contact and a lowering of EE in the family.

How secure are these findings? The EE measure was originally developed in Britain, but has now been used in a number of countries, both in the developed and in the developing world. These studies are summarized in Table 2.2 (some of the more recent studies are of preliminary data, but the definitive findings are unlikely to differ much). All in all, they add up to quite an impressive consensus about the value of the measure in predicting

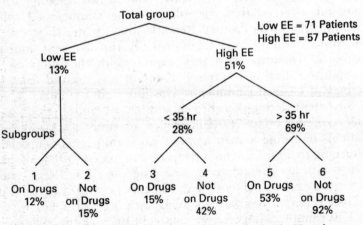

Fig. 2.1 Relapse rates at 9 months (taken from Vaughn and Leff, 1976).

Table 2.2 Results of prospective studies of EE

Author:	Date	Location:	No of Subjects	Episode:	Follow-up:	Relapse rate High EE	Low EE
Brown et al.[1]	1962	S. London	97 (male)	All	1 year	56%	21%
Brown et al.	1972	S. London	101	All	9 months	58%	16%
Vaughn and Leff	1976	S. London	37	All	9 months	50%	12%
Leff and Vaughn[2]	1981	S. London	36	All	2 years	62%	20%
Vaughn et al.	1984	Los Angeles	54	All	9 months	56%	28%
Moline et al.[3]	1985	Chicago	24	All	1 year	91%	31%
Dulz & Hand[4]	1986	Hamburg	46	All	9 months	58%	65%
MacMillan et al.	1986	N. London	67	First	2 years	63%	39%
Nuechterlein et al.[5]	1986	Los Angeles	26	All	1 year	37%	0%
Karno et al.	1987	S. California	44	All	9 months	59%	26%
Leff et al.	1987	Chandigarh, India	76	First	1 year	33%	14%
Tarrier et al.[6]	1988	Salford, England	48	All	9 months	48%	21%
Parker et al.[7]	1988	Sydney, Australia	57	All	9 months	48%	60%
McCreadie & Phillips	1988	Nithsdale, Scotland	59	NA	6 months	13%	11%
					12 months	17%	20%
Barrelet et al.	1988	Geneva, Switzerland	41	First	9 months	32%	0%
Budzyna-Dawidowski et al.	1990	Cracow, Poland	36	All	1 year	32%	9%
					2 years	72%	18%
Ivanovic & Vuletic	1989	Belgrade, Yugoslavia	60	All	9 months	64%	7%
Mozny	1989	Rural, Czechoslovakia	68	All	1 year	60%	29%
Cazzullo et al.	1989	Milan, Italy	45	All	9 months	58%	21%
Stricker et al.	1989	Munster, W. Germany	99	All	9 months	high EE sig worse	
Ferrera et al.	1989	Madrid, Spain	31	All	9 months	44%	38%
Vaughan (pers. comm.)	1989	Sydney, Australia	87	All	9 months	52%	23%

1. Their measure of 'emotional overinvolvement' was the prototype of EE.
2. Follow up of same patients as Vaughn and Leff (1976).
3. Non-standard criteria for high EE
4. An unknown number of subjects were not living with their EE rated relatives.
5. All patients on fixed dose fluphenazine.
6. Patients receiving standard care with or without education in the authors' intervention programme.
7 All relatives were parents. An unknown number of subjects were not living with parents at the time of readmission or reassessment.

relapse, although the amount of time relatives spend together has only shown up as an important factor in studies carried out by the original group of British workers. Some of the studies do fail to find an association between EE level and relapse, but these are in a minority, and in some cases have serious failings. We have discussed this research at greater length elsewhere (Kuipers and Bebbington, 1988; Bebbington and Kuipers, 1991).

If EE is a robust predictor of relapse, the relapse rate of schizophrenia should be affected by anything that affects EE. One example is the different organization of family life in many Third World countries in comparison with the industrialized West. Extended families are the norm in the former.

The better course and outcome of schizophrenia in developing countries is well established (WHO, 1979): could it be the result of different family characteristics reflected by the EE measure? Wig and his colleagues (1987a) carried out an EE study in the area around the Indian city of Chandigarh. As expected, relapse rates were low, particularly in the rural areas. Despite this, there was still an association between hostility expressed by relatives and subsequent relapse a year later. This suggests that the good outcome of schizophrenia in this culture might indeed be the result of beneficial family structures and traditions (Leff et al., 1987). In other words, both in Chandigarh and in London the relapse rate appears to be related to EE, but it is lower in India. This could therefore have been due to the lower levels of EE in India. Loglinear analysis of the pooled Indian and London results (Leff and Vaughn, 1976a; Leff et al., 1987) suggested that the better outcome in India can be entirely explained by lower levels of EE and that the effect is of considerable strength (Kuipers and Bebbington, 1988). So, not only does EE have predictive value across very different cultures, it may also serve to explain differences in outcome of schizophrenia in those cultures.

However, Hogarty (1985) has recently raised an important point, arguing that EE only predicts relapse in men, not women: this seems to have some support from the available evidence (e.g. Vaughn et al., 1984). Brown and his colleagues (1972) did claim that EE was equally predictive for male and female sufferers, but, even so, EE may be of less clinical significance in women because the prognosis is relatively better for other reasons (Salokangas, 1983). The question of the role of EE in female patients remains open.

Finally, it must be remembered that the value of EE is not confined to schizophrenia. The measure has now been found to be useful in a variety of other conditions, including depression (Vaughn and Leff, 1976a; Hooley et al., 1986), bipolar disorder (Miklowitz et al., 1988), anorexia (Szmukler et al., 1987), mental handicap (Greedharry, 1987), Parkinson's disease (MacCarthy, pers. comm.), inflammatory bowel disease (Vaughn, pers. comm.) and senile dementia (Bledin et al., 1990). While much theoretical and clinical interest remains in the use of EE in schizophrenia, the measure itself appears to tap difficulties common to the care of many disabling problems. High EE ratings have also been noted in the key workers of long-term patients with schizophrenia (Watts, 1988).

How does an Adverse Home Environment Lead to Relapse?

It has always been assumed, not unreasonably, that the home environment characterized by high EE represents a form of psychosocial stress. How then is relapse mediated? One possibility is that it operates via physiological arousal.

There is now quite a lot of evidence from psychophysiological studies in line with this suggestion. Patients seem to be physiologically aroused when with high EE relatives, but not with low EE relatives (Tarrier et al., 1979, 1988b: Sturgeon et al., 1984). Indeed, Tarrier and Barrowclough (1987) demonstrated a differential psychophysiological effect in a man living with one high and one low EE parent, depending on which was present. The arousal provoked by critical relatives seems to be nonspecific, and has been observed in disturbed (non-schizophrenic) adolescents (Valone et al., 1984).

However, despite changes in EE due to a successful social intervention programme (Leff et al., 1982), there were no concomitant changes in psychophysiological ratings of patients, which turned out to be related to relapse independently. In other words, the benefit from changes in EE does not appear to work through changes in levels of arousal. This research has been reviewed in more detail elsewhere (Kuipers and Bebbington, 1988; Turpin et al., 1988).

Leff and his colleagues (1983) have incorporated these ideas about arousal into an overall model of relapse in schizophrenia, using material from their intervention study to strengthen their argument. They concluded that patients unprotected by medication might relapse in response to *either* a life event *or* living with a high EE relative, but that patients taking medication required exposure to both factors before they would relapse. In this model, medication operates generally to raise the threshold for the psychosocial provocation of relapse, suggesting that life events and EE might have a common mechanism.

What Does EE Pick up about Families?

For historical reasons, the Expressed Emotion measure is a bit of a mixture. It covers two attributes of relatives that at first sight seem distinctly different. It would seem reasonable to regard criticism and hostility as similar, and distinct from the other attribute of EE, that is, emotional overinvolvement. Criticism is seen frequently in both the spouses and the parents of those with schizophrenia, whereas spouses are less likely to be overinvolved than parents. Can these two aspects of EE be regarded as inherently distinct, and if so in what sense?

Some authors (e.g. Koenigsberg and Handley, 1986) are very keen on the principle of keeping them distinct. There may well be differences in their associations: for instance, emotional overinvolvement may be particularly associated with poor premorbid social functioning (Brown et al., 1972; Miklowitz et al., 1983). However, Tarrier and his colleagues (1988b) failed to distinguish between the two patterns of behaviour from the patient's psychophysiological responses to the presence of a relative. Moreover,

emotional overinvolvement, they show a similar ability to predict alone (Brown et al., 1972; Vaughn et al., 1984; Leff et al., 1987). Thus, although the attitudes look very different and may have different origins, they may actually work in the same way. Hooley (1985) argues that both criticism and overinvolvement are strategies reflecting a need to control situations. Is emphasizing these similarities useful? We think that it is probably good to retain some separation of the two ideas for clinical reasons; as we suggest in later chapters, emotional overinvolvement and criticism may require different therapeutic strategies.

In the research studies, it has become traditional to dichotomize EE levels into high and low groups. This may be a reasonable thing to do, inasmuchas the presence of critical comments above a certain level perhaps identifies a qualitatively different home environment. However, this is something of a stab in the dark as it has never actually been demonstrated. The danger of using EE in this categorical way is that it may lead to over-rigid attitudes towards intervention with relatives in routine clinical practice. We know from our own experience that there are clinicians who think it necessary to ask for an EE rating before feeling they should offer a service to families. This rather misses the point.

EE uses an individual relative's behaviour at a single time to predict the likelihood of a subsequent relapse in the schizophrenic patient with whom that relative lives. All well and good, but what does EE actually mean in terms of the interplay between members of the patient's family?

It has always been presumed that the measure is predictive because it indicates either some continuing feature of the interaction between the relatives, or their capacity to deal with crises (Kuipers, 1979). From early days, it was known that relatives who made frequent critical comments when interviewed alone would behave similarly in the presence of the patient, albeit more restrained in the second setting (Rutter and Brown, 1966; Brown and Rutter, 1966).

There is now further evidence for the generalization of the relative's behaviour. Miklowitz and his colleagues (1984, 1989) and Strachan and his colleagues (1986) have used the *affective style* coding system developed by Doane and her colleagues (1981) to assess families taking part in a standardized task designed to recreate interaction in a laboratory setting (Goldstein et al., 1968). Negative affective style in these direct interactions is consistently highly correlated with EE measured in the usual way. Hubschmid and Zemp (1989) have shown that high EE relatives engender a more negative emotional climate, a conflict prone structure, and more rigid patterns of interaction.

Kuipers and her coworkers (1983) also found it possible to distinguish between high and low EE relatives in family interviews. During discussions that included the patient, high EE relatives talked for longer and were poorer listeners than low EE relatives. MacCarthy and her colleagues (1986) have recently found that highly critical relatives appear to provide an unpredictable home environment for schizophrenic patients. Greenley (1986) has shown that high EE is associated with fears and anxieties on the part of relatives, particularly when they did not attribute the patient's behaviour to illness. Preliminary results of a study of attribution in the relatives of schizophrenic patients suggest that causal beliefs are systematically related to the relatives' emotional characteristics. The more critical and hostile relatives tended to attribute negative outcomes to causes that were more idiosyncratic to and controllable by the patient (Brewin, pers. comm.)

A study of depressed spouses throws further light on the behavioural counterparts of EE. Hooley and Hahlweg (1986) reported sequential analyses of interaction patterns between 44 couples where one partner was depressed. They found that high EE couples had a varied but largely negative style of interaction. Low EE spouses typically had a continuous positive exchange. It was also possible to distinguish between the high and low EE samples on levels of warmth, hostility and marital satisfaction.

There is now evidence that high EE is associated with less effective coping responses (Bledin et al., 1990; MacCarthy pers. comm.). High EE carers of demented elderly people used strategies such as distraction, avoidance, overeating and denial, rather than more positive approaches like problem-solving and seeking social support (Bledin et al., 1990).

Birchwood and Smith (1987) have a primary interest in describing and quantifying families' coping behaviour and coping styles. They investigated the relationship between these characteristics of relatives and the outcome of schizophrenia in terms of relapse, social adjustment and psychopathology. Although it overlaps with the previous EE research, their work provides new data on family behaviour in this situation. Clearly the link between the relative's ability to cope with the problems of living with someone suffering from schizophrenia and the affective style of their interaction with them is a crucial issue: the causal direction is unknown, but probably complex. It is a pity that these studies have been developed independently of any EE assessment, although the authors' current research does include it. Indirectly, their examples add to the evidence that poor coping in relatives overlaps with high levels of EE.

Interestingly, when the patients' own responses are examined, those living with low EE relatives give vent to significantly fewer critical statements and more autonomous statements than those from high EE families. In other words, criticism is reciprocated. This finding is independent of the level of symptoms experienced by the patients (Strachan et al., 1989).

Thus there is now good evidence for thinking that EE represents an aspect of ongoing family interactions. As we argue in Chapter 5, this does not mean at all that most families rated high on EE are appreciably deviant. The characteristics of their interaction are subtle, and it is only because they seem relevant to outcome that they are a proper topic of interest to the clinician.

Nevertheless, identifying the less adaptive coping responses, and assisting relatives to change them for effective strategies, may enable clinicians to feel more at ease in helping families.

One of the problems of EE is that the interview and the skill of rating take time to learn. At present, many clinicians seem to think that, without the benefit of an EE rating (which is unlikely to be available), they are not in a position even to try to help relatives. They therefore often want to know short-cuts to the recognition of the family at risk. This cannot be done without loss of information that may sometimes be important. However, even low EE families have a range of needs, so that falsely dichotomizing them in terms of their requirements for treatment may be counterproductive. This would certainly be the case if the low EE rating is of a type liable to change under stress (see p. 37). It is possible that the assessment of coping responses may be a more accessible way of finding out what sort of help a family needs with its difficulties.

Researchers have hardly ever related levels of EE to the 'burden' experienced by relatives, although as we have seen in Chapter 1 the literature on the latter is now substantial. It seems likely that relatives with high levels of EE will find the same behaviour more burdensome than those who are low on EE. This is also probably related to coping styles. Bledin and his colleagues (1990) have recently shown that high levels of strain, EE, and maladaptive coping strategies tended to be associated in those caring for demented elderly persons.

The Origins of Family Attitudes Towards a Mentally Ill Relative

The EE measure therefore probably reflects a variety of attitudes and behaviours characterizing the family's response to a mentally ill relative. What is the origin of these characteristics? On the evidence so far available, they do not appear to be closely related to the severity of the patient's disorder, although it is possible that poor premorbid social functioning has a particular capacity to elicit overinvolvement. Birchwood and Smith (1987) have raised theoretical objections to EE. They argue that the original workers were wrong in thinking that EE reflects some enduring trait of relatives, and that the measure actually picks up an emerging attribute. In other words, high EE is something that develops as the response of some relatives to the burdens of living with someone who has schizophrenia. This argument is based on the fact that high EE is less apparent in relatives of those experiencing first rather than subsequent admissions for schizophrenia. There is certainly a lower relapse rate in first admission (33%) when compared to subsequently admitted patients (69%) (Leff and Brown, 1977), although there are alternative explanations for this. Moreover, recent work has suggested that at least some components of high EE are associated with abnormalities of various sorts in the patient (Miklowitz et al., 1983; Mavreas et al., 1990). However, the causal direction is as usual unclear.

Birchwood and Smith (1987) therefore present a feedback or adjustment model, whereby families' coping efficacy and coping style, along with other predictors such as the quality of family relationship, will develop over time.

In a sense, Birchwood and his colleagues have attacked something of a straw man. It must be virtually axiomatic that the characteristics of high EE arise from an interaction between the attributes of relative and patient.

The value of EE assessment may be crucially related to the fact that the relative is dealing with the upheaval surrounding the patient's admission to hospital. In time the disturbance settles, and a sizeable minority, perhaps a quarter, of high EE relatives become less critical (Brown et al., 1972; Dulz and Hand, 1986; Hogarty et al., 1986; Tarrier et al., 1988a; Favre et al., 1989). Initial assessments have therefore focused on the admission period. Low EE relatives tend to stay low, although Tarrier and his colleagues (1988a) did report a minority who changed to high levels. There is relatively little other evidence as to the stability of EE measures over time. In the studies of Leff and his colleagues (1982, 1985), the high EE control group showed no significant overall changes in EE over the intervention time of nine months, although two of the twelve relatives did spontaneously become low EE.

It seems possible that there are three groups of relatives: at one extreme, there are the very low EE relatives who cope well whatever the circumstances. At the other extreme are very high EE relatives who have multiple problems, and cope badly with most of them, including the patient. In between seems to be a variable group who may change category spontaneously or through the intervention of others, depending on their ability to learn new coping skills, and to use them in surmounting crises. If the new skills are insufficient, they may display reduced EE at one assessment, but revert back when there is a crisis which they are unable to manage (see Fig. 2.2).

This idea has recently received some confirmation in a study of the stability of EE over a nine month period in 35 relatives of 22 patients with schizophrenia (Favre et al., 1989). They found stable high and low EE relatives, but also a proportion of unstable relatives who typically displayed fewer critical comments (6–10) than the stable high EE group. The authors noted that the relatively few changes oberved in EE levels seemed to depend on factors *other* than the clinical state of the patients.

The hypothesis that high EE reflects one of several adverse environmental stresses (Day, 1986), which may trigger a schizophrenic episode in vulnerable individuals (Zubin et al., 1983; Liberman, 1986; Wing, 1987) remains the most plausible model of its effects. There are still gaps in our knowledge of mediation: of how high EE is perceived by the patient, and of how the stress is translated into florid symptoms. It may be that schizophrenic patients who are less able to cope with these particular social

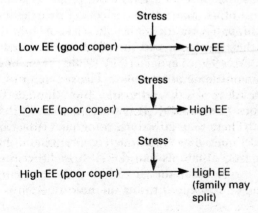

Fig. 2.2. Patterns of EE over time.

stimuli are those who are most vulnerable — unable to process information effectively because of their cognitive defects, they allow themselves to become overloaded (Hemsley, 1987). This would fit the data on social contact from the British studies, but it may be that those patients who do not work out adequate avoidance strategies are also the most impaired. Those with over-involved relatives have been shown to be the most impaired socially (Birchwood and Smith, 1987) and may be most at risk, either because of their intrinsic problems or because an over-involved relative is harder to get away from ('she follows me everywhere').

To Blame or Not to Blame?

As we suggested above, the change from the more ambitious early social theories of schizophrenia to the more restricted versions exemplified by the EE research is really one of relative emphasis: current social theories certainly hold that relatives have an influence on the manifestations of disorder. How then can the imputation of blame be avoided?

Here we must keep firmly in mind the distinction between empirical causation and moral responsibility. Unless they are recklessly inconsiderate, we only hold people to blame when the consequences of their actions are both intended and repre-hensible. We cannot in justice blame them for the unintended results of their behaviour. In general, the relatives of those who suffer from schizophrenia are no more prone to act in bad faith than the rest of us, and adverse effects of their actions arise by and large through ignorance. They do not know how their actions will affect their relatives, and therefore cannot foresee bad con-sequences. Moreover, even if they could, they might not be able to frame rational alternatives. The problems of living with schizophrenia are of a different order from those encountered in ordinary social intercourse. It is thus quite likely that attempts to cope with them may go wrong, sometimes disastrously so. In consequence, relatives may through ignorance and inadvertence create domestic situations that do not help either themselves or the patients with whom they live. This does not seem to us to be the occasion of blame, but rather an indication for offering them help.

The inherent injustice of blaming relatives is however only one ground for avoiding it. An equally good reason is that it is plain counterproductive. Relatives are well aware that difficulties at home may not be the ideal environment for someone who is fragile and vulnerable to symptoms of mental illness. They are only too ready to blame themselves for this state of affairs, and this makes them sensitive to the possibility that others blame them too. If they feel that this happens when they see the professionals concerned with the care of their sick relative, they are quite likely to be touchy and to shun further contact even if this is the only pathway to help for their difficulties. It is hard to gain the confidence of relatives under these circumstances, and strategies for dealing with this crucial issue are dealt with at length later in the book.

The training of doctors puts them at a particular disadvantage when faced with relatives. First, they rarely receive specific instruction in dealing with them. Secondly, the concept of 'consultation' primarily concerns a relationship between patient and doctor. This confrontation is assumed to be confidential unless clearly specified to the contrary. In consequence, doctors tend to be a bit cagey with relatives. While they may sometimes see them as important sources of information, they are themselves sparing of the information they give. Such a view of the ethics of consultation must seem primitive and counterproductive to any one who is conscious of the reciprocal repercussions of individual health and family relationships. It is also unnecessary, as it is quite possible to respect confidentiality by negotiating what may not be revealed rather than what may be.

These aspects of medical training compound the inappropriate wariness of psychiatrists dealing with their patients' relatives. There is certainly no doubt that many psychiatrists behave in this way. This is clear from studies that have canvassed the opinions of relatives about their mutual meetings.

Other members of the multidisciplinary team may be less tentative about involving themselves with the families of their patients. However, relatives rarely seem much happier with the service from other staff members.

We are convinced that this state of affairs must change.

3·Intervention Studies

Once it became apparent that particular attributes of family interaction might have a deleterious effect on the course of schizophrenia, intervening to change these attributes became a logical next step. Several reports of social intervention with the relatives of patients with schizophrenia have now been published, and others are nearing completion. Intervention studies are important both clinically and theoretically.

The theoretical significance of these studies emerges from what they imply about the causal role of family atmosphere in provoking relapse. There are occasional contrary findings from the prospective studies listed in Table 2.1, and some obvious gaps remain in our knowledge of mechanism. The critics of EE research must however contend with the generally positive results of intervention: the ability to change outcome by changing family atmosphere is highly suggestive of a causal link.

The London Study

Leff and his coworkers (1982) looked specifically at 'high risk' families, i.e. those who demonstrated high levels of EE and were also in high mutual contact. All patients were maintained on medication, but while the control group (N=12) had standard hospital care, the experimental group (N=12) were offered a package consisting of education sessions at home, a relatives' group to which both high and low EE families were invited, and sessions at home that included both the family and the patient. The aims of these interventions were to reduce either the EE levels of the relatives, or mutual social contact to less than 35 hours a week. One of the aims was achieved in 75% of the experimental families (9/12), and there were no relapses in these families in the nine months following discharge from hospital. Overall the experimental group showed an 8% relapse rate (1/12), contrasting with 50% (6/12) in the control group, a value exactly in line with expectation. Critical comments, a major component of EE, were significantly reduced only in the experimental group, which also showed reductions in emotional over-involvement that failed to reach significance, probably because of the small numbers. A two year follow up (Leff et al., 1985) revealed that, *for those patients who remained on medication*, there was a 20% relapse rate in the experimental group versus a 78% (7/9) rate in the control group. However, two subsequent suicides in the experimental group mean that, overall, 50% (6/12) of patients relapsed in the experimental group, compared with 75% (9/12) in the control group, a nonsignificant difference. The suicides, which occurred some time afterwards, appeared to be related to intervening changes in circumstances, not to the intervention itself, and were in families where the experimental aims had not been achieved.

The First Los Angeles Study

Falloon and his colleagues (1982) chose a sample of 36 parental families, most of whom were rated as high EE, but a few families were included because of high levels of 'tension'. All patients were again on maintenance medication. The control group (N=18) had the best 'standard care' available, consisting of individual treatment that took up an amount of time comparable to that received by the experimental group. Thus, this study controlled for the 'attention only' effects of treatment. The experimental group (N=18) received education sessions and family intervention at home. The latter was based on a family problem solving approach, and consisted of a structured attempt to delineate problems and enable the family to come to some consensus.

The results were similar to those of the previous study: in the nine months of follow up, the control group had a relapse rate of 44%, the experimental group one of 6%. These workers also reported reduced family burden. Although they do not comment on whether EE was changed significantly, a reduction in 'negative affective style', particularly of criticism and intrusiveness, was apparent in the experimental group as therapy progressed, and was strongly associated with the reduced relapse rate (Doane et al., 1986; Goldstein and Strachan, 1986). Negative affective style is closely related to ratings of EE.

The two year follow up (Falloon et al., 1985) once more suggests that the effects of family intervention are enduring.

By 24 months, 83% of their control patients had had a major relapse of schizophrenia, contrasting with 17% of the family treated patients. The families in the experimental groups also reported less subjective burden (Falloon and Pederson, 1985). The experimental group complied more with medication, and this could possibly have confounded the effect of the family intervention (Strang et al., 1981). However, the levels of medication overall were lower in the experimental group than in the control group, so this cannot vitiate the significance of the findings greatly.

The Second Los Angeles Study

Wallace and Liberman (1985) compared social skills training of the patient and behavioural family therapy with a treatment package of individual and family therapy that was much less focused on individual problems. Twenty eight male patients, all on neuroleptic medication, from families with at least one high EE member were randomly allocated to each treatment. The specific treatment group had a better relapse rate at nine months follow-up (21% cf 50%), but this difference, although suggestive, was not significant. Unfortunately, the effect of the type of family intervention cannot be separated from that of the type of individual therapy in this study, and no data are given concerning the effects on relatives. This sort of intensive and focused intervention may have a place in the management of schizophrenic patients recovering from an acute episode, but there might be considerable problems in applying it to those with fewer assets or more chronically disabling symptoms.

The Pittsburg Study

Hogarty and his colleagues (1986) have reported a large trial of social treatment and medication in the prevention of schizophrenic relapse. They had a sample of 134 parental high EE families, of whom 90 accepted all the treatments. They divided them into four groups: family treatment and medication (N=21); social skills and medication (N=20); family treatment, social skills and medication (N=20); and drugs alone in a standard dose (N=29). The family treatment consisted of an education workshop followed by sessions at home. The aims of the latter were to increase information about the illness, to augment social networks and reduce isolation, and to offer help in coping with problems. The social skills training was aimed at helping patients to improve their social perception and to be more assertive with their families. This was conducted with the patients alone.

The authors reported no relapses over the next year in the family treatment/social skills/medication group, whereas the family treatment/medication group had a 19% relapse rate, the social skills/medication group had a 20% relapse rate and those on drugs alone had a 41% relapse rate. The social skills training appeared, therefore, to add significantly to the effectiveness of family treatment. They did not count minor episodes responding to treatment in two to three weeks as 'relapses', and this may make the study less comparable with the other studies. This study aimed to lower EE in the families, albeit indirectly, and it is therefore interesting that good outcome in the treatment condition was not necessarily associated with a reduction in EE.

The first Los Angeles study and the Pittsburg study both suggest that intervention not only reduces relapse rate but also improves social performance (Hogarty et al., 1986; Doane et al., 1985). This is almost certainly an important factor in the reduction of family burden.

The Hamburg Study

There has also been an intervention using separate relative and patient groups (Köttgen et al., 1984). This differs from the other studies because it had a younger patient group, a more analytically oriented approach, and no separate education input. The nine month relapse rate was 33% in experimental high EE families versus 50% in control families. This result suggests that groups organized along these lines are less effective. Strachan (1986) has argued that the psychodynamic group treatment may have been overstimulating, and the absence of a focus on practical problem solving may not have been beneficial either.

The Salford Study

Another well-conducted intervention study has just been completed in the Manchester area (Tarrier et al., 1988a; Tarrier and Barrowclough, 1987). Sixty-four patients from high EE families were randomly allocated to one of four groups. One group received only routine hospital treatment, and the second was in addition given a short programme of education. The third and fourth groups also received a behavioural intervention. Nineteen patients from low EE families were randomly allocated either to a routine treatment group or to one given the education package in addition. Treatment and assessment dropouts were included in the analyses, so the results give a conservative impression of efficacy. All patients were prescribed medication, mostly in depot form.

The aims of the behavioural intervention were twofold; first, to lower EE through changing the relatives' style of coping: secondly, to improve the patients' level of functioning through the identification of needs and the planning of goals.

The results showed a significant and equivalent effect for the behavioural interventions, but no observable effect of education on its own. The behavioural interventions were successful in reducing both EE and relapse rate. Indeed, the effect on EE was reflected in significant decreases in both critical comments and emotional overinvolvement, the latter possibly more evident because of the large sample size. Moreover, the effect on relapse appeared to be mediated via the effect on EE. Critical comments also decreased somewhat in the routinely treated high EE group. There were also significant albeit inconsistent effects of the intervention on social functioning.

The differences between the treatment groups could not be accounted for in terms of compliance with medication or of amount of contact with standard psychiatric services.

The Second London Study

A further study by Leff and his colleagues (1989), comparing education plus family treatment with education plus a relatives' group, is now complete and suggests that both treatments can be equally effective. All patients were maintained on neuroleptic medication. However, it was harder to engage relatives in the group than to treat them in their own homes: Eleven out of twelve families accepted family therapy, only six of the eleven families took up the offer of the family group. Only one of the patients from the therapy group families relapsed, and only one of the patients from families who actually attended the relatives group. Three patients relapsed from the five families who declined the relatives' group. Low relapse rates were clearly associated with reduction in EE.

The Sydney Study

A study from Sydney is also now complete (Vaughan, pers. comm.). The intervention was carried out only with relatives, and 34 patients were divided equally between experimental and control groups. All relatives were rated high on EE, but not all were in high contact. The focus of the intervention, comprising 8–10 sessions of at least one hour, was on the behavioural analysis of current problems and the examination of attitudes. At nine month follow up, 7 of the 17 patients in the family counselling group and 11 of the 17 in the control group had relapsed, a non-significant difference. EE status at follow up was assessed in only 12 patients, so little can be said of the impact of the counselling process on EE. A possible explanation for the high relapse rate in both groups is that around half the patients did not persist with medication, thus making the effect of intervention hard to demonstrate.

Uncompleted Studies

Family interventions in schizophrenia are now becoming big business. The current and very large National Institute of Mental Health collaborative study is designed to examine the effects of various drug regimes and two types of family management: 'applied family management', drawing from a behavioural perspective after the manner of Falloon and his colleagues (1982), and a less directive 'supportive family management', comprising communication, sharing of problems, and support. Each group of patients attends an educational workshop. Although this project will add to our knowledge of management in schizophrenia, the assessment procedures do not include EE.

A study currently being conducted in Hamilton, Ontario (Monroe-Blum, pers. comm.) is comparing the effectiveness of social skills training for the patient and a family intervention very similar to that of Leff and his colleagues (1982), both separately and in combination. The social skills training is very intensive, and is directed at specific social problems. The patients to be included in the study are selected on the basis of long-standing (more than five years) illness without recent exacerbation. Relatives will be assessed for EE, which will be used to stratify the patients before allocating them to the treatment groups.

It is obvious from these studies how relevant the EE research has been to the provision of a structure within which effort can be focused on specific treatment aims and interventions evaluated. This seems likely to account for at least part of the success of these programmes: it has been relatively easy to demonstrate change, and it has been possible to attain the limited and specific goals of the interventions.

However, each study described so far has been very much a specialized attempt, using a highly motivated clinical and research team to investigate a novel intervention. The application of the results in a routine way to the work of a busy clinical team must be the next phase. Some idea of the possible applicability of these techniques can be gleaned from Table 3.1. Around 60% of patients with schizophrenia live with relatives, and of these from 40–70 live in high EE households. Moreover, patients tend to return to the family home as their illness persists.

Studies of Intervention within Ordinary Clinical Services

Two studies aiming to bridge a gap by introducing to ordinary clinical practice the techniques of intervention developed in the course of research have now been published. The first offered an intervention suited to the needs of the very long-term mentally ill (MacCarthy et al., 1989; Kuipers et al., 1989). This provided relatives with a minimum intervention, carried out by two members of the clinical team. This comprised education and a monthly group. The sample of patients was taken from the team's case load; most but not all had been given a diagnosis of schizophrenia, and there was a range of EE levels among the relatives. Four relatives (23%) declined to take part, in two cases for good practical reasons, and the other relatives attended the group for about a year. Results showed a reduction in EE in the relatives of the experimental group, together with improved coping skills. Symptomatic relapse rates were low in both experimental (22%) and control (23%) groups of patients, linking in with evidence that reducing disability may be more relevant and more feasible in this long-term sample than the prevention of relapse (Liberman, 1986). Patients in the experimental group did indeed show significant improvement in social functioning. This model of intervention would seem at first sight to be practicable, acceptable and cost-effective in a wide range of facilities.

Table 3.1 The applicability of the EE measures

	Location	Proportion of patients living with a relative	Proportion of relatives rated high on EE	Proportion of households rated high on EE
Brown et al. 1962	S. London	60%	NA	52%
Brown et al. 1972	S. London	NA	NA	45%
Vaughn and Leff 1976	S. London	NA	NA	49%
Vaughn et al. 1984	Los Angeles	NA	NA	67%
Moline et al. 1985	Chicago	NA	NA	70%
MacMillan et al. 1986	N. London	60%	53%	NA
Karno et al. 1987	Los Angeles (Mexican-American)	NA	28%	41%
Wig et al. 1987	Aarhus	NA	NA	54%
Leff et al. 1987	Chandigarh	NA	23% 30% urban 8% rural	23%
McCreadie and Robinson, 1987	Nithsdale Scotland	63%	43%	42%
Tarrier et al. 1988	Salford England	NA	73%	77%
Parker et al. 1988	Sydney Australia	NA	NA	74%
Barrelet et al. 1990	Geneva Switzerland	NA	NA	66%
Vaughan, pers. comm.	Sydney Australia	NA	NA	53%
Rostworowska pers. comm.	Cracow Poland	NA	NA	70%

In a very different setting, McCreadie and his colleagues (1990) evaluated a package of treatments offered by professionals working in an everyday NHS setting in rural Dumfriesshire. The package included educational seminars, relatives' groups and family meetings. The groups focused on day-to-day problems of coping with schizophrenic relatives.

Of 63 relatives approached, 32 refused and 14 of the remainder attended neither the educational seminars nor the relatives' group. There were no differences between attenders and refusers in terms of EE status, gender or relationship to the patient. However, the relatives who refused were significantly less likely to live with patients who had relapsed recently. Seven of the 17 relatives who received the whole package were rated low on EE.

The intervention made no difference to the number of people who relapsed in an 18 month follow-up period, but did tend to reduce the frequency of relapses. No change in EE was observed following the intervention. The relatives themselves were pleased to have taken part and found the experience useful.

This study differs from most in the field as it concerned schizophrenic patients in remission and living in the community (Bebbington, 1988). This makes it difficult to extrapolate results to more usual client groups. It does emphasize the problem of engagement — although the relatives' commonest reason for declining the intervention was 'things are fine at the moment', any sense of pride seemed mixed in with a sense of resignation and resentment.

What do the Intervention Studies Tell Us?

A number of issues arise from this review of the recent literature.

One of the theoretical purposes of interventions with high EE (and high contact) groups is to cast light on the causal significance of the family environment in engendering relapse. The success of some interventions has been associated with their effectiveness in reducing EE, contact or negative affective style (Leff et al., 1982, 1989; Falloon et al., 1982), and the less successful interventions of Köttgen and her colleagues (1984) and of McCreadie et al. (1990) did not manage to reduce EE. This suggests that high EE may indeed be a marker of a family environment that adversely affects the course of schizophrenia. However, in the Pittsburg study (Hogarty et al., 1986), good outcome in the combined treatment group did not require reduction in EE. There are other reasons for reserving judgement on the causal role of the family environment. Many studies have involved small numbers, and it remains possible that, when interventions include working with patients, reductions in EE are secondary to improvement in their behaviour, rather than due to primary and beneficial changes in the behaviour of the relatives. However, the study of Tomaros and his colleagues (1988) is somewhat against this interpretation, as direct improvement of negative symptoms and social function by vocational training and social therapy had little effect on family atmosphere, at least in the short-term. The results of the interventions, taken together with the impressive consensus from the predictive studies, therefore form a strong indication that EE may indeed reflect a causal process.

Clarification of this issue requires longitudinal study of the stability of EE and its relationship to relapse in a large sample. We need to know how changes in EE relate to changes in the patient.

While having different aims and orientations, the successful interventions so far completed have displayed several common themes:

1 There is a positive attitude towards the families. This entails acknowledging that problems are real and difficult, and that relatives have positive resources that can be utilized, but not exploited, by the therapists (Kuipers and Bebbington, 1985).

2 Importance is given to education. This has not actually proved useful in changing the attitudes of high EE relatives by itself. However, it seems vital because of its interaction with later components of intervention. It provides a model for co-operation, and for sharing information between relative and clinician, thus creating a sense of optimism (Berkowitz et al., 1984). It also encourages families to engage in treatment, by offering them what they want and letting them get to know the professionals they will later work with.

3 Interventions have tried to deal with the current problems of the families, and how they can negotiate a solution or adopt different methods of coping. A focus on limited treatment aims appears to be very useful in starting the process off, as the achievement of small realistic goals can set a new pattern.

Successful interventions have tried to help relatives and patients (usually both) to deal with stress, to improve competence and social interaction, and to increase understanding, tolerance and empathy.

4   Several of the interventions (Wallace and Liberman, 1985, Hogarty et al., 1986, Monroe-Blum, pers. comm.) have included a social skills training (SST) element. This is not social skills training in the accepted meaning of the word (Falloon, Argyle) as it does not address global deficits. The SST used in the intervention studies is directed at dealing with fairly specific problems of a social nature. The results of social skills training directed at deficits in skill rather than dealing with specific situations have not shown impressive results in schizophrenia (Shepherd, 1986; Liberman et al., 1987). The value of a more focused variety of SST has been emphasized by Shepherd (1988) as a way of escaping the persistent difficulties of generalizing improvements in patients with longstanding disorder. This is also in keeping with the problem solving approach with other family members. The techniques of social skills training as described in some detail by Anderson and her colleagues (1986) would seem an appropriate adjunct to the style of working with families advocated in this book. The preliminary evidence suggests that the two approaches may work synergistically (Hogarty et al., 1986).

5   Social treatment works best against a background of effective neuroleptic medication. Given that the patients are often at great risk of relapse, the discussion of medication may be a crucial first stage in helping the family and the patient to begin the process of understanding problems and coping with them.

6   Interventions of this type are not particularly time-consuming, in comparison either with standard treatment, or with the time spent in dealing with emergencies that would otherwise arise more frequently. Several research studies have compared the amount of staff time devoted to preemptive interventions with families with standard hospital care. Falloon and his colleagues (1982, 1985) found that their intervention took up an amount of time commensurate with that used for the standard hospital management, but with much better outcome. Leff et al. (1982) worked out that their extra input averaged less than 2½ hours of staff time per month per family.

The issue of what is the best type of intervention and who should be targetted remains to be clarified. It seems likely that a range of interventions will be developed to suit the needs of different families. However, some general lessons may be taken from the intervention studies carried out so far.

The general consensus favours some kind of education package as a preamble to more focused intervention. There is also considerable agreement between research groups that the best technique for intervening with family members is behavioural problem solving (Spivak et al., 1976). The degree of structure and the rigidity of application differs, but the underlying principles seem common to all. Facilitating problem solving by families with mentally ill members is a high level skill, and one that runs counter to the training of many therapists. One possible explanation for relatively unsuccessful interventions is that the therapists lacked this particular skill in some degree (McCreadie et al., 1990). This is not unlikely in the current situation, in which researchers worldwide are stumbling towards the specification of effective family management with very few guidelines (whatever they may claim afterwards!). However, we are now beginning to tease out the key elements in intervention, and the latest studies are now able to rely on manualized treatment procedures (Monroe-Blum, pers. comm.).

Much less agreement exists about the context of intervention. Some researchers have relied heavily on family problem solving sessions with single families (Falloon et al., 1982, Hogarty et al., 1986, Tarrier et al., 1988a). Others have used groups of relatives (Leff et al., 1982, Kuipers et al., 1989) and still others, groups of relatives and patients together. We are not too keen on the last option, but in general it is likely that different contexts will be appropriate for different families according to circumstances, and the correct decision will be fairly obvious. We discuss the issues with reference to those with longstanding illness at greater length in Chapter 4.

Part Two
Techniques of Intervention

4·Strategies of Intervention

The aims of intervention in the long-term group can be clearly specified from the research on social factors and from the range of problems faced by these particular patients, their relatives and the clinical staff looking after them.

The first aim is to help patients manage their illness so that they have as few residual disabilities as possible, and operate in as normal an environment as is practicable. This is the standard aim of rehabilitation programmes for the long-term mentally ill.

The second is to enable carers to understand the range of problems that beset patients, to help them deal with their own emotional turmoil, and to facilitate a constructive set of coping responses. Relatives need to understand something of the process and complexities of mental illness, to be able to contain their criticism of patients and to transform it into a more constructive approach. Carers often need specific support for the range of emotions that they will go through in response to the illness. They may need further help with feelings of overinvolvement that seem to result from a translation of the perceived needs for help and support on the part of patients into their own need for control. In consequence, they provide high levels of caring which are only appropriate for the acute stages of illness, and which later on may easily impede recovery and patients' attempts at independence.

From the viewpoint of clinical staff, interventions must be seen to be feasible and practicable, and to have a fair chance of success. It is helpful for dedicated personnel if some beneficial changes can be seen as a direct result of all the effort that they put into patient care. One of the difficulties of working with the long-term group is that success is often partial and rarely obvious, and it is therefore valuable to make clear at the beginning of an intervention what is to be counted as a change for the better.

It is important to enable staff to fit an intervention into part of their routine: suggesting that they should add to their already considerable work load is not likely to be translated into action. The approaches suggested here do not require that staff should do more, but that the contacts they already have with carers and patients are utilized more effectively, and with clear aims. Some aspects of intervention, say a relatives' group, may well reduce workload by enabling one or two staff members to see several families at once. Overall, the research evidence is very encouraging: interventions that do not necessarily take longer or require more intense involvement than standard hospital care are able to minimize the rate of admission to hospital, to reduce the likelihood of crisis, and to improve the quality of life of patient and carer. In the longer term, they thus reduce demands on services. For instance, if patients have had a crisis admission to hospital under the powers of the Mental Health Act in each of the last five years, an intervention that manages to prevent this over the next couple of years will at the very least provide a breathing space for them and their relatives. Equally important, it will provide a stable period during which a start can be made on recovering lost skills and developing a greater independence on both sides. Moreover, the cost in hospital personnel and facilities will have been considerably less. Emergency action and the occupation of hospital beds are after all extremely expensive. Even if there is another relapse after this, the very fact of a longer gap between admissions can be used as a way of restoring the confidence of patients and their families that some improvement is possible.

The information we have at the moment suggests that these aims should be implemented in a way that takes account of certain basic elements. These are, first, that an attempt is made to provide information to relatives. All the successful intervention programmes so far have offered education to carers. There have been a variety of formats, and by itself education does not seem very good at what it purports to do, that is, improving the relative's knowledge. However, it does seem to engender optimism and it is clear that it facilitates the engagement of carers in later stages of treatment. Presumably it has face validity: after all, it means that professionals are at the very least doing what carers endlessly request — being prepared to listen, to answer questions and to share their knowledge and their ignorance, rather than retreating behind a barrier of defensiveness and suspicion, perhaps disguised as an adherence to confidentiality.

It may be that another clear pointer to the style an intervention should take is provided by the Hamburg study (Köttgen et al., 1984). Their psychodynamic approach with families was not successful in changing outcome, quite possibly because schizophrenic patients can find such techniques disturbingly intrusive. We would argue that a step by step pragmatic approach, aimed at solving the problems that trouble carers and patients, is more likely to be useful.

Finally, reducing relatives' criticism (intolerance and mis-attribution of symptoms, particularly negative ones) and over-involvement (inability to lead relatively independent and adult lives and treating patients as children) is a crucial aspect of successful intervention, and will be discussed in detail in succeeding chapters.

There is no consensus about the way to satisfy these aims, and it seems likely that different approaches may be equally successful, provided they embody the principles outlined above. There is therefore scope for teams and individuals to decide which method will best suit local conditions, including the organization of services and their own needs and interests. Flexibility and adaptability is after all one of the hallmarks of effective work with long-term patients. This leaves it open for those involved to develop services that work both for staff and for patients.

Engagement

One of the obvious features of patients with longstanding mental illness and their relatives is their reluctance to engage with the psychiatric team (Kuipers, 1983). By the time patients have been ill for several years, disillusionment with services is likely to have set in very firmly. After all, not many people would choose to deal with psychiatric hospitals, staff, day centres and the rest if they could decently manage to get on without them. Some families do indeed try to cope on their own, although they usually end up making (often unsatisfactory) contact again later on. Having to let outsiders into intimate details of family life and history, particularly if they do not actually appear prepared to give much in the way of help, is one of the many understandable reasons why carers and patients may be less than enthusiastic about offers of assistance.

The starting point must therefore be that families are likely to be reluctant, and many are also evasive, angry, ungrateful, and critical of our best efforts. An offer of assistance is an explicit suggestion that family members are not coping through their own efforts; that they are doing something wrong. A desire for help is therefore alloyed with a dislike of public admission of failure. Staff must be very aware of these conflicting emotions in any initial approach, and prepared to handle the tendency towards negative responses tactfully and sensitively, without retaliating or being rejecting.

It may be helpful to think of approaches towards relatives in a similar light to those directed towards patients. This is not to suggest that carers necessarily resemble patients. They normally have rather more in the way of resources, and these can be tapped by a constructive approach, similar to that used with patients who are much less disabled by their mental illness than those we deal with in a long-term setting. The aim is to establish a true partnership that involves all participants in an effort to deal more effectively with each other, whether carer, patient, or staff member. The professionals involved, who are after all not likely to be living with the patient and therefore have time away from them, have a clear obligation to show the tolerance and helpfulness they are trying to encourage in carers. It is easier for staff to set this sort of example than for relatives to follow it, but without it there is little prospect of improving relationships.

The exhibition of tolerance and willingness to help is part of a more general requirement of staff that is of crucial importance: a positive attitude towards families. Bennett has suggested that all staff working with this long-term group of patients have ideological reasons for their commitment, whether religious, political or humanitarian (Watts and Bennett, 1983). For those who wish to deal with the family as a system, it is important that their reasons for working in this area do not interfere with the development of a positive attitude towards relatives. It is not possible to work with families in this way, if you really think that they are totally to blame for patients' problems, or are very unpleasant people. Such opinions are very quickly picked up by relatives who, already feeling guilty and unable to cope, are sensitive to imputations from professional staff. One mother said 'they told me it was all my fault, and she should go and live in a hostel. But they never did anything about it, and she came back to live with me'. This sort of interaction only increases bitterness and recrimination between staff and carers, even if the relative's interpretation of it is distorted. The ideal is to avoid the occasion for unhelpful distortions in the first place.

We therefore advocate a positive and persistent approach by staff, particularly in the initial stages of intervention. If it is difficult to gain access, with appointments broken or refused, this should be accepted as commonplace, an indication for attempting new arrangements rather than giving up in irritation. Difficulties of engagement do not predict failure in the later stages of treatment. Vigorous outreach with these groups, both patients and carers, is an aspect of management that is known to be useful and acceptable.

Offering education can be an ideal way of creating the conditions for successful engagement, as it is often what relatives say they want. Moreover, it does not make great demands, either of staff or of relatives. Nor do relatives see it as threatening even in the context of what may feel like a very explosive or intolerable situation.

Models of Service Delivery

Table 4.1 sets out several models of delivery with which we are familiar. Other combinations are conceivable and may be feasible. We think that a psychiatric team should ideally be able to offer different styles of service to different clients according to need. The type of provision can be arrived at following negotiation with clients and their families. The models are certainly not mutually exclusive, and if one set of elements is not acceptable, another combination can be offered. Models 2–5 all contain an educational component, and it is therefore appropriate to discuss the format of this component.

Education

By itself education does not change EE attitudes or outcome (Cozolino et al., 1988; Tarrier et al., 1988b). Indeed, it leads to very small changes in the amount of knowledge carers have about psychotic illnesses (Berkowitz et al., 1984; Smith and Birchwood, 1987). Thus we do not discuss models showing education without additional input.

However, all these approaches have improved optimism and engagement in subsequent therapy, so education does appear to

Table 4.1 Possible modes of intervention for families of the long-term group

	Education + relatives group	Education + home visits to family	Relative only support group	Patient counselling
Positive effects	low staff cost	hard to avoid (for family)	offers support	Individual problems addressed
	reduces relatives' isolation	deals with individual family problems in detail	no staff cost	standard staff cost
	offers support			
Negative effects	some drop out	high staff cost	may not enable change	relatives not offered service
	does not deal with all problems	isolation not changed		
	patient may feel excluded			

have an important function in setting up the process of intervention. The best way of offering it has not been established. Varying styles have been tried in the experimental studies: one day workshops, with several families at a time (Anderson et al., 1986), didactic sessions at home, with or without written information (Leff et al., 1982, 1989; Falloon et al., 1984; Barrowclough et al., 1987), an interactive session using a questionnaire (MacCarthy et al., 1989), and relatives' groups with a didactic structure (Smith and Birchwood, 1987).

The content of this education has not been standard either, but it usually consists of some relatively straightforward attempt by the professionals to explain what we know, and what we do *not* know about these illnesses, to discuss issues of diagnosis, cause, and pharmaceutical and social treatments, and to examine ways relatives can influence outcome (Leff et al., 1987; MacCarthy et al., 1989).

There is also dispute about the format, with some therapists using quite sophisticated audiovisual aids. In our view a relatively informal approach with a structure which is more apparent to the clinician than to the relatives does just as well, and allows an easy exploration of the families' concepts and beliefs. This can then be used as the basis for modifying their views and extending their knowledge. There is evidence that using the actual belief systems of relatives in this manner is the most effective way to get information across (Tuckett, 1982). It can be supplemented with leaflets or advice about books on the subject.

For the long-term group, the diagnosis itself may not be such an issue, as carers are likely to have heard the words schizophrenia, or manic depression, or psychosis from some clinician over the years of contact with mental health services. However, it is often the case that mere provision of a diagnosis does not inform them, and that their understanding of its implications and their own ability to affect outcome may be very limited. Thus education is still relevant for this group, even if they may seem to have been given information before.

A related point is that it takes considerable time to take in information, particularly if it is unexpected, unwelcome, out of keeping with the views already held by the relatives, and given at a time of crisis when the ability to concentrate and comprehend is at its lowest. Our knowledge of the poor efforts at communication made by most health professionals (Tuckett, 1982), combined with the relatives' lack of receptivity, makes it very likely that exactly those carers who most need to understand that much of the problem behaviour is due to an illness called schizophrenia are the hardest to convince.

Certainly we have found that it is sometimes extremely difficult to shift ideas about causality; it is natural to seek explanations for our experiences, and most carers will have developed their own views about the origins of patients' illnesses. Because we as professionals can never be definite about causes in the individual case, we may not be in a good position to change these ideas. Carers who have convinced themselves the problems started because of a motorbike accident, a fall from a window, or a girlfriend leaving, are not likely to alter their views, particularly if they have been left to develop them over several years. However, actually naming the set of behaviours as an illness, as something recognizable and not that unusual, is reassuring in itself and also gives hope that perhaps something can be done.

Thus for the long-term group, it is crucial to give relatives enough time to take in the required information. This means not one session, but several, and ideally the information should be repeated frequently over several months. The detailed content of the information appears less important than the manner of its delivery. Because of their requirements for evaluation, all the intervention studies have used standard methods. However in our view, it is actually *answering carers questions*, in an open and sympathetic way, and *continuing to do so whenever required* that is one of the most important aspects of any educational approach. In our experience, carers will quite often come along to do just this — ask a variety of questions — and this is usually despite previous talks with psychiatrists involved in their relatives' care. It appears that this helps them to mull over information that at some level they have already been given, as part of the arduous task of assimilation. Such assimilation is particularly difficult when attitudes and reactions have become very entrenched, rigid and pessimistic.

Offering information is thus quite a skilled task, requiring from staff sympathy and the patience to cope with the same questions repeated many times over months of contact. Done well, it provides a pattern for the development of a relationship of trust between relatives and staff. Typically carers will say 'oh, we were never told that', or 'no-one said that before, we never knew it was called....'. This has happened even when we had ourselves given carers a formal education package including diagnostic information just a few weeks previously. This does not indicate stupidity or obtuseness on the part of relatives (or of staff), but that such information is very hard to take on board. This is probably true of most novel information, particularly when it requires carers to try something new.

The exact ground covered by the information provided seems, as we say, to be less important. The day-long workshop used by Anderson and her colleagues (1986) goes into very considerable detail about the aetiology and neurobiochemistry of schizophrenia. In our view this may be too much: although Anderson and her colleagues tie in a great deal of what they teach with problems the family is likely to face, there still seems considerable redundancy. The information given does require to be accurate, up-to-date and related closely to the problems of the particular patient. The topics we tend to cover are listed in Table 4.2. Various aids are available; the National Schizophrenia Fellowship produces a leaflet (Leff et al., 1988), and Birchwood provides a series of booklets. Our book '*Living with Mental Illness*' (Kuipers and Bebbington, 1987) appears to have been useful to relatives interested in more extensive information.

Table 4.2 The provision of information to relatives

Diagnosis
Have the relatives been given a name for the illness?
Is it in line with the diagnosis in this patient?
If so, what do they understand by it?

Causes
A short and appropriately pitched account of the possible biological and social factors influencing the emergence of disorder. Emphasis on the imperfect status of our knowledge.

Symptoms
What do they understand of the symptoms of the disorder?
Talk them through the positive and negative symptoms.
Emphasize the way the disorder can influence behaviour.

Treatment
The range of treatment available.
The function of medication; side effects.
Importance of social treatment: structure; calm atmosphere; careful schedule for progress; idea of fragility, if carer not already aware of it.

We think it is important to give a name to the disorder as far as possible. Although, as we discuss in Chapter 5, there have been worries about labelling, in our experience a sympathetic discussion and exchange of information does not itself add to the stigma of mental illness.

Where possible, we have found it helpful to see people in their own homes for this stage of the intervention. A home visit emphasizes that the professional cares — has made an effort — and is more comfortable and relaxing for the recipients than an appointment in the strange surroundings of an office at the hospital or health centre. However, not all carers welcome a home visit initially, so flexibility is required about the venue, as with all aspects of intervention.

So far we have been discussing the offer of education primarily to the carers. This follows the actual development of these approaches in the research studies of intervention, as they were originally provided just after the patient had been admitted to hospital. At a time when patients were usually acutely ill, it was more appropriate to talk to the carers by themselves. This practice has been maintained over the years, as there are advantages in seeing carers without the patients. Many relatives feel constrained by the patients' presence. In consequence, discussions under these conditions are not as forthright as may be necessary.

However, patients also have a right to information, and staff have an obligation to provide it. In our experience it is best, particularly in the long-term group, to give information separately to relatives and patients. Patients may lack insight, temporarily or permanently, and disagree that there is anything the matter. Dealing with this lack of insight while also trying to help carers adjust to a new model often leads to muddle and confusion. The style of transmitting information requires to be tailored to the capacities and existing beliefs of the recipient, and it may need to be different for relatives and patients. Thus, the two sides should if possible be seen separately. If this cannot be managed, the information will probably have to be given in smaller packages and over a longer time scale.

Informing carers is only the first stage in the process of altering their situation. The information then must be used to help carers change in three specific ways. These are, first, to begin to understand and become more tolerant of behaviour that is mainly due to the illness itself; secondly, to become more realistic in their expectations of change; thirdly, to have a proper perspective of the probable time scale of change. This last requirement is particularly important for those whose relatives suffer from illnesses likely to be of long duration.

Model 1 — relatives' self help groups

The advantages of these are that they are usually already available in the locality. They require no staff time as, by definition, they run independently of professional staff (apart perhaps from occasional invited input). They provide local social networks and support, and reduce feelings of isolation, stigma and shame. They may also energize carers into playing a more active and constructive role with other relatives if they wish. The best self help groups can also enable new members to understand and change their approach to patients, and help them manage their many problems more constructively. In the UK, the National Schizophrenia Fellowship and the Manic Depression Fellowship are the two best known and reputable agencies organizing such groups at present. The NSF also has a number of very helpful information leaflets, and provides a telephone support service.

The disadvantage of a self help group is that many relatives will not attend. It takes considerable motivation and courage to attend an unknown group, and many carers do not feel able to take up what is on offer locally. It may also require access to transport unavailable to relatives in straitened circumstances. There is little evidence that self help groups can themselves enable carers to change their responses to patients, and indeed, unless they are exceptionally well run, this would seem unlikely. Finally, patients may feel excluded.

Model 2 — education plus facilitated relatives' groups

A facilitator is someone outside the group — normally a member of the professional staff — whose function is to enhance the group process. Good facilitators should enable groups to use constructively the opportunity of sharing experiences, discussing common problems, and agreeing some solution or way of coping. They will also assist group members to express emotional distress and anxieties without feeling threatened or vulnerable. Being outside the group allows facilitators to be objective and help the members focus on their common problems rather than avoid or deny them. It does *not* mean that facilitators should not empathize with and care about the very difficult and upsetting problems that group members may have to deal with.

As its best, the combination of educational sessions run by professionals and a facilitated group of this type can help reduce the stigma, isolation and loneliness often found in carers of the mentally ill, whose social networks may be almost as restricted as those of the patients (Anderson et al., 1984). It has the advantage of considerable cost effectiveness as one or two staff members can see up to ten families at a time. In our own study, even a group meeting only once a month was able to show significant benefits to participants, that is, for a mere three hours of staff time per month (Kuipers et al. 1989). Once a month is also quite an appropriate interval when patients have longstanding problems unlikely to change suddenly. This sort of interval is usually an acceptable time commitment for the participants, both staff and relatives, while remaining effective. Where patients are more acutely disturbed with a greater danger of crisis, more frequent meetings will be needed, perhaps once a fortnight (Tarrier et al., 1988a,b; Leff et al., 1989). In the long-term group, however, our experience suggests that most crises can be anticipated by the monitoring provided by a monthly group, as both carers and staff will be adept at recognizing signs of trouble. It has also been demonstrated that this model is capable of changing coping patterns, of reducing EE, and of improving outcome in patients (Tarrier et al., 1988a,b; Leff et al., 1989; McCarthy et al., 1989).

However it shares the disadvantage of self help groups, in so far as not everyone can or will attend. Motivation cannot be guaranteed and may have to be enhanced. The use of facilitators may be crucial here, as they can make themselves known to carers before their first attendance at the group. This is particularly so where facilitators are also responsible for conducting the preliminary education sessions at home. The obvious 'giving' of professional time and trouble can then be 'repaid' by attendance at the group, which once started will often be continued for its own sake. However, some carers cannot attend because they are physically disabled; one relative was agoraphobic and never left the house. Even offers of transport may not necessarily solve these problems. Other carers may find the scheduling of the group inconvenient: whatever time is chosen, some people will find it difficult. We have tended to have groups in the afternoons: many relatives are retired, and others do not work for other reasons. However, those who do work then have to make special arrangements. Evening groups do not suit women or the elderly, who feel unsafe out at night in our inner city area, particularly in the winter.

The other consideration is that not every carer can cope with attending a group. After all, group meetings require a certain level of social and cognitive skill which not all relatives possess. One carer who had previously abused alcohol was left with severe memory deficits, and although he attended the group on a few occasions it was clear he was unable to participate in a useful way. Because in the long-term group about 10% of carers will have been or remain in receipt of psychiatric care themselves, they may well have difficulties of motivation or concentration that make group attendance unlikely to be successful. In the study of Leff and his colleagues (1989), only 50% of potential carers attended, and this obviously reduces the viability of this method.

Finally, groups may not be able to cater for all needs. Group members who are atypical in some way, such as being the only spouse present, or young, or the relative of a patient with many neurotic symptoms, may find that others do not share their problems and then feel less able to participate. In addition, very shameful or worrying individual problems, such as child abuse in the family, are usually unsuitable for discussion in a group setting, and must be tackled elsewhere.

Patients may also feel excluded by a relatives' group, although, in practice, we have found that apart from an occasional patient whose illness involves strong feelings of persecution, most are quite able to accept the carers' need for help and to talk to other carers about the problems they face.

Model 3 — Education plus family problem solving sessions

The obvious advantage of this model is that it is much harder for families to avoid! Home visits by staff, initially for education sessions and later for the intervention stage, establish a pattern that only requires family members to stay around at the times scheduled for visits. This does not necessarily guarantee attendance of course, but it certainly makes it more likely, and disabled or housebound carers can then be included. The time for the family meeting can also be individually arranged to suit most participants.

Problem solving sessions at home allow therapists to deal with intimate and individual problems that might not ever be raised in a more public group setting. Domiciliary family sessions of this type include the patient, and thus allow a much more interactive approach to be used.

Patients' views and goals can be canvassed directly, and they can in consequence be involved in setting targets and negotiating contracts, rather than having them more or less decided in their absence. The presence of patients allows more direct modelling by the therapist of appropriate ways of listening to them and interacting with them. This can be particularly helpful if the patient is habitually dismissed or described very negatively by carers: 'he's like a vegetable' or 'she only talks rubbish'.

There is clear evidence that education and family problem solving work well to improve outcome (Falloon et al., 1982; Hogarty et al., 1986; Leff et al., 1989).

The disadvantage of this model is that it is more time consuming, and consequently more expensive. It usually involves two staff members having to set aside time for travelling to and from the family home, as well as the time given to intervention. Transport costs of staff will be particularly high in rural areas, and in any case this assumes that some transport is available. Home visiting on public transport can be extremely time consuming, even where a suitable service exists. These costs might be justified for families with very difficult individual problems, motivational or transport difficulties, or in a setting where home visiting is routine. Staff shortages may also cause problems, for example in a team where staff participation in home visits leaves a day facility understaffed.

The other main disadvantage is that individual home visits do nothing to counteract the isolation, the sense of stigma, and the feeling that no-one else has these problems so typical of long-term families. This may make it harder to facilitate change, as feelings of resignation and pessimism may be entrenched. In a group setting in contrast, there is a range of difficulties, and one carer's progress can be used as a catalyst to encourage others to attempt something new.

Model 4 — education, family sessions and a relatives' group

As has been discussed, this combination of elements has the advantage of being effective even for those families who are poor group attenders, and can maximize the assets of each approach. If families are willing to participate in all the components, the frequency of each can be reduced; family meetings can supplement the relatives' group, or vice versa, so that overall the family is contacted, say, once a month.

Model 5 — patient skills training

In order to maximize the effectiveness of management, direct intervention with the patient should normally be routinely incorporated into attempts to involve carers. However, in some cases it is not possible to engage relatives, and it is then important to attempt to change family patterns indirectly by working with the patient. On its own, this is a model of last resort.

The Pittsburg study showed the positive effects on patient outcome of 'social skills' training. This was a specific attempt to help patients become more assertive in the family setting, enabling them to state their views and to discuss problems without it leading to destructive arguments and stalemate (Anderson et al., 1986).

On a more general level, individual work with patients to enable them to cope better with an overstimulating or over-involved family setting may well be sensible. Helping patients to recognize triggering situations and discussing strategies such as limited withdrawal or clear limit setting can certainly ease distressing family relationships. One patient learned to withdraw temporarily from her husband's shouting matches. Previously she had joined in, but this had always made her symptoms much worse, and certainly solved nothing.

In families where carers do not engage in treatment, either refusing or dropping out soon after starting, this may be the only approach. Some patients refuse to let staff 'bother' the family. One man insisted that his mother would be upset by phone calls or other contact with staff. These refusals have to be respected of course, unless relatives themselves make contact, whereupon staff may be able to proceed further.

The disadvantage of this model is obvious: carers themselves are offered no support. It goes back to a more traditional model of working just with the patient, although with the specific aim of enhancing coping within the family setting.

Stages in the Process of Coping with Mental Illness in Relatives

While weighing up the likely impact and costs of a particular model, it is worth considering the stage that families have arrived at in coping with the patient's illness.

Adapting to this kind of long-term trauma follows a course that has considerable parallels with the process of coping with other traumatic situations, such as bereavement or the affliction of a relative with other long-term handicaps such as physical illness or mental handicap. For the purpose of clinical guidance, it is useful to distinguish stages in these adaptation processes, and we feel that there are advantages to a similar identification of stages in the adaptation to severe mental illness in a relative. Although there is probably less consistency in the way relatives of the long-term mentally ill pass through these stages, with some being omitted entirely by some relatives, staging has particular relevance for strategies of engaging the relative in the process of management.

We would first identify an *initial stage* of shock and upset when patients first come to notice, often the time of first admission to hospital. This is the first and public realization that something is wrong. However, this stage of shock and upset may continue for years, with increasing levels of anger, and denial of the fact of mental illness or the unlikelihood of cure. Second opinions may be sought at much cost and difficulty — relatives may shop around continually for a better service or a cure. Any degree of recovery is seen as the beginnings of a return to normality, and considerable frustration and helplessness may result in carers and patients, who cannot understand why recovery from the acute illness does not equal a return to normal participation in society. This stage is exacerbated by professionals who do not explain what is happening and assume that the family either is not very involved, or for some reason does not need to know.

A *second stage* can be distinguished by the advent of some degree of realization. This is associated with relatives constructing a view of their situation which is consistent, but often idiosyncratic. Relatives at this stage will often have acquired at least some kind of diagnostic and clinical information, although this may have been provided inadvertently, inconsistently, and obscurely. It is therefore not surprising that it may be absorbed inaccurately. Indeed, this transmission of information may be spread over several years, and may even have been changed from time to time. As is obvious from looking through casenotes of long-term patients, the diagnosis is often changed, ranging for example from personality disorder through manic depressive illness to schizophrenia, schizo-affective disorder, and chronic schizophrenia, and back to obsessive personality. Carers typically register the diagnosis but do not understand what it means. The result is often frantic searches in libraries for inappropriate information on the 'Jekyll and Hyde' personality. They usually find nothing that ties in with the behaviour of their own loved relative, and so they decide themselves on some explanatory fiction, such as 'nervous breakdown' or 'lazy' or 'needing a job'. This stage is usually associated with some adaptation in lifestyles, and both patients and relatives recognize that life will never return to normal. However, the price paid for this adaptation is that both sides by this time also feel very pessimistic about the future. Most of the contact with professional staff may be taken up with arguments about medication, seen by both patient and carer only as a negative element, bringing unpleasant side effects and no apparent benefits.

A *third stage* can then be entered, characterized by a further deterioration in relationships between staff, carers and patients. Staff see as unreasonable the constant demands of carers for new medication or for admission, or for help with patients' physical complaints. The relatives in turn feel that staff are unhelpful, obstructive and even rude. Emergencies arise, and are often badly handled by the staff; the police may be involved, case notes go missing, the various members of the clinical staff make inconsistent decisions. Patients may stagger from one crisis to the next, often maintaining in the interval between emergencies that there is nothing the matter. This situation may also last for years; typically in this stage staff members try to pass the family on to other services, and the difficulties are compounded by the involvement of new agencies unaware of the previous input, or by more and more people from different agencies trying to sort things out in incompatible and counter-productive ways; one family of ours managed to involve in quick succession local social services, a Salvation Army officer and a psychiatric registrar in a hospital 200 miles away.

The *final stage* is that of coping and effective adaptation. This may never be reached, but ideally it should replace stages 2 and 3 and be entered immediately after the shock and upset of stage 1, but before anger and denial set in. In this stage, patients and their families begin to tackle problems and cope with the difficulties. This does not necessarily depend on professional help; indeed, as things stand with many psychiatric services today, carers usually have to manage it for themselves. We know, for instance, that patients who have repeated crisis admissions are a minority of the long-term mentally ill.

In this stage, carers realize that 'something is the matter' and that 'it does no good to argue'. In other words, they face up to the fact in all seriousness that the patient is in trouble and not able to respond as usual, and they are then able to adapt their own approaches to maximize and maintain recovery. 'I learnt to be more patient' said one mother. This realization is usually independent of the provision of a formal diagnosis or clinical guidance, but seems to emerge from the carers' own careful observations, leading to the conclusion that the patients' behaviour is altered and to some extent no longer under their control. The reaction may, indeed frequently does, encompass the sorrow and upset seen in other stages, but relatives are able to build on this a constructive approach which helps both them and the patients to cope. Patients and their relatives may only contact professional staff infrequently, and this is more likely to occur at unavoidable crises, such as the illness or death of the carer.

In our view, this staging of potential responses is important because the style of intervention should be informed by an appreciation of the stage reached by the family in question. The aim of intervention is to ensure that families end up in something that looks like the final stage described above, but with the greatest degree of adaptation and integration that can be achieved.

Stage 1 families, particularly if the situation has gone on for years, need the diligent and continuing provision of information. This is augmented if they attend a group, as this greatly assists the realization that their problems are not unique and that they may be confronted effectively. Individual family sessions should be offered (usually at a later stage) where they are needed to deal

with specific issues such as modelling more appropriate behaviour towards the patient.

However, many long-term patients and carers will be in Stage
2. Some progress and adaptation will have been made, but not in
a very consistent, coherent or constructive way. The emotional
atmosphere is most likely to be one of pessimism, combined with
criticism of patients' negative symptoms. These families often
benefit most from the provision of education and family sessions
in which patients are included. A relatives' group can be offered
concurrently or, perhaps more effectively, as a follow up.

Stage 3 families are rather used to dealing with professional
staff and are often dismissive of new contacts. Families like this
require a very flexible approach from staff, who should be ready
to offer one or more of a range of facilities depending on their
ability to engage. The main purpose of education may be tangential, providing the possibility of changing the relatives' view
of services by showing that staff are willing to put themselves out
to help the family, and appear to believe that such help is worthwhile. This may shift, albeit ever so slightly, the family's pessimism, both about the clinical services and about their own
situation. Once it has been possible to engage the family seriously,
most of the difficult work of change and adaptation will follow in
family and group sessions. In stage 3 it is helpful to improve
consistency by cutting down the numbers of staff involved. In
order for families like this to take seriously the offer of help and
to feel that they will not be rejected (again) by staff, it is necessary
to offer a long-term involvement (over years). This may mean
being taken on by senior members of staff, who are less likely to
move on. By implication the staff then also give the message
that the family and patient are worth working with in the long
term — this may be the first sign of hope for them.

If the family has reached the final stage through their own
efforts, it is known that they may still be beset by problems of
isolation, stigma and loneliness and by external crises. A relatives' group may be a particularly useful facility for such families,
a place to share problems and a means for them to widen their
social contacts. Even low EE relatives who cope well are known
to benefit from such group experiences (MacCarthy et al. 1989).

5·Reducing Criticism

'He never got up, *never* got up, till late in the morning' (a mother speaking of her son).

Criticism — Lay and Technical Usages

In some ways it is a pity that the term *criticism* has been adopted as the name for one of the component ratings of the expressed emotion measure. It has led to considerable confusion. The term indicates a very specific phenomenon: it must be made quite clear that when people use the word criticism in common parlance, they seek to convey something very different from this technical meaning.

When in the ordinary way people are described as critical, it is usually because they are seen as expressing appreciable distaste, dislike or hostility towards others. However, such clear signals rarely form the basis of the rating of a *critical comment* in the course of the Camberwell Family Interview. These ratings are not primarily derived from the context of the remark, but rather from extremely subtle changes in the emphasis, tone, and pace of speech. This is why EE assessments cannot be made of transcripts, only of tape recordings. As such they pick up a range of emotional qualities from slight irritation or unhappiness about some action or situation, all the way through to real dislike, intolerance and frustration. In practice, this means that the carer is giving a relatively subtle indication of their feelings about the patient and how their tolerance and patience is not endless.

The generation of critical comments must be spontaneous, that is, they do not comprise direct responses to questions. There must be at least some unforced amplification, and they often emerge as relatives spontaneously move to another topic. It usually requires a degree of rapport on the interviewers' part before relatives will give vent to critical comments. Most people will deny negative feelings if asked about them directly, as they are aware of the social unacceptability of expressing them.

One of the techniques in the Camberwell Family Interview is to enquire about examples. While direct questions are used, and are necessary for factual ratings, the affective components picked up in the CFI are more likely to arise when respondents feel free to describe a recent incident. Critical comments often emerge as the relatives paint a picture of some particular occurrence in their relationship with patients. This emphasizes the subtlety of the rating and the behaviour on which it is based. Much of this is likely to be lost in an ordinary clinical interview with its more direct style, and the tendency by interviewers not to follow up tangential remarks.

Only the end of the range of critical comments is equivalent to the lay use of the term critical, and at this point it merges with the CFI measure *hostility*. This is actually met fairly infrequently in the relatives of those with schizophrenia, even in those rated high in EE. Misunderstanding of this issue is responsible for some hostility towards EE research, which is erroneously believed to be saying very negative things about the patients' relatives. This is not so (and even in cases where a high EE rating indicates that relatives are handling their situation less than well, this would not in any case be, in our view, the occasion for blame — see p. 38).

Many whose knowledge of the topic is limited to reading the research literature think that high EE ratings mark out relatives who have rendered their family situations catastrophic. Again this is rarely so. It is much more likely that they are responding to the common and almost inevitable difficulties attendant on living with someone with a severe and persistent mental disorder, with consequent tendencies to misattribute and misunderstand what is going on. These cannot be seen as unexpected, wrong or abnormal responses. Most people would behave similarly in a corresponding situation. It is only because of the empirical evidence that critical comments are predictive of outcome and relapse in schizophrenia, that it is worth trying to analyse the details of what the relatives do, and to modify their approach if this is possible. The imperfections of these relationships would hardly be the concern of clinicians, if one party to them had not been made vulnerable through a susceptibility to schizophrenia.

Where then are critical comments directed? In fact they can be aimed at almost anything, and relatives differ greatly in what they mention, in the same way that people generally show great variation in what they find annoying. Criticism of the ill relative may be tangled up with other criticisms, for instance, of the hospital and its services, or of other members of the family, so the focus may not be restricted to the patient.

Criticism encompasses remarks both about the behaviour and about the personality of mentally ill relatives. In some cases, relatives focus on bizarre behaviour, for example:

> 'When he was living by himself, it was back to square one, everything *over* the place; he eats and just throws it on the ground, although there was a dustbin; the butter, it fell on the floor, he didn't pick it up; it was all over the carpet, all over everything' (a mother of her son).

> 'When he's not on medication he'll just *sit* there hallucinating: you can't get through to him, really, but he never admits that he is, not once' (a mother of her son).

It is more usual for negative symptoms to be mentioned, and as we have pointed out before, these are more often misattributed because of the considerable overlap with normal behaviour.

> 'He wouldn't wash unless you told him, and even if you told him, he'd say 'yes all right', but he wouldn't *do* it .... and then you'd have to tell him *again*' (a mother about her son).

One does not have to have schizophrenia to lie in bed in the mornings or to be careless in disposing of cigarette ash. Many relatives who make critical comments report that in their view the patient has always behaved in the way they now complain of and that it predated any question of illness. 'He never got up, did he, never got (out of bed) up till *late* in the morning' (a mother about her son). Thus two thirds of the critical relatives in Vaughn's study thought that the patients' behaviour was due to their personality:

> 'He never could get up in the morning even as a teenager; it's even worse now'; 'he's just awkward, unemployed, not bothered about anything'.

This emphasizes the failure of correct attribution, quite clearly apparent to the clinician and now receiving corroboration in the research literature (Brewin, pers. comm.). Relatives find it difficult to disentangle what is intentional, and what is not about the patients' behaviour. In some cases, this leads them to make criticisms of the patients' moral character, and it is at this point that the relatives' attitudes tip over into what non-professionals mean by the word critical, but which is technically defined as hostility in the ratings of the CFI.

Criticism in the EE sense is much more common. Most families make one or two critical remarks, particularly at times of crisis such as a hospital admission when feelings are running high, and more easily and frankly expressed. Although for the purpose of formal rating criticism can be clearly defined, the actual training of staff to recognize Critical Comments reliably takes time and motivation. Considerable interest has therefore been expressed in alternative methods whereby criticism could be recognized more easily by practitioners, thus avoiding the need for formal training. Although such informal recognition will always be fallible, research studies, together with our own clinical experience, provides a few obvious pointers.

As we have indicated, we now have some evidence from research studies of what criticism (as defined in the CFI) means in terms of the relationship between patients and relatives. High EE relatives engender a more negative emotional climate, a conflict prone structure, and more rigid patterns of interaction. Their attempts at coping are often maladaptive. Critical relatives tend to put their viewpoint over forcefully, to listen less to patients, and to be dismissive of positive aspects of their behaviour. Moreover, criticism is reciprocated: patients living with high EE relatives give vent to more critical statements and fewer autonomous statements. These attitudes on the part of relatives also have a direct effect on the coping style of patients so that either they retaliate, leading to tension and arguments, or they withdraw, with a consequent reduction of a range of behaviours. In family meetings, withdrawn patients are likely to remove themselves physically or mentally from this upsetting over-stimulation.

However, in general the CFI picks up very subtle gradations of behaviour, and our knowledge of the interactions represented by it must be far from complete. So, although relatives still voice critical comments when they are interviewed together with the patient, they often do so much less frequently. This is partly because they often recognize such remarks as socially less acceptable when made in front of patients, but it is also the result of a realization that it is not helpful to make such comments in their hearing.

If critical relatives do suppress their criticism to a large extent in the presence of patients, how is it that the interaction has such a notable effect on relapse rates. Again this is likely to be the result of subtle nuances of manner that probably colour the relatives' whole approach to patients. Although they may feel they are doing the best they can to help patients, the latter, from the nature of their condition, are particularly sensitive. In consequence, relatives need considerable help in fundamentally reconsidering their situation and the way they should respond to it.

The characteristics of criticism in the EE sense therefore have implications for the manner of clinical intervention. From what has been said it is clear that clinicians should be prepared to spend time with relatives on their own, and also allow them space in which to voice their concerns. This can then be the basis of a complex process of re-education based on the analysis of current situations.

Criticism often and understandably appears to have its origins in failure at some level — it is closely connected with the carers' frustration at not being able to sort out problems. Carers have usually tried all the normal repertoire of coping responses — persuasion, listening, nagging, ignoring, physical encouragement — and have found them unsuccessful. An illness like schizophrenia, which has many bizarre and unusual features, requires new coping responses that are not part of the normal repertoire. Unless carers have realized this, the frustration and anger brought on by repeated failure to change or improve things is very quickly transferred onto patients. This is particularly the case in a competitive, individualistic culture like ours, where it is assumed that adults take responsibility for their own behaviour. Failure to manage adult roles — not being able to go to work, refusing to look after children or do housework — can arouse particular resentment. In schizophrenia of course even more fundamental problems can arise: self neglect, refusal to get up, wash, or dress in clean clothes, declining all responsibility over money.

Misunderstanding the nature of the symptoms of severe mental illness is often central: relatives misattribute the behavioural components of symptoms to factors other than illness, frequently ascribing them to enduring personality features. Problems viewed as arising from unwillingness rather than disability will be blamed on patients' 'laziness' or 'selfishness': 'he was just being pigheaded' as one mother said. Relatives misapprehend other things as well, notably the nature and effects of pharmacological and social treatments.

Hostility

Hostility, certainly in our culture, is the extreme end of the criticism range. It is rated essentially from the content of the remarks made during the CFI, although it almost always shares the tonal and emphatic qualities that go to make up the ordinary critical comment. It tends towards a criticism of the person as a whole rather than of a specific instance of a disliked action — generalization is implicit in this rating. This reflects a quite radical process of misattribution. At its most extreme, it is expressed in remarks that are unequivocally rejecting. For example:

> 'I almost hoped he would get run over. That would be better than the person dying and yet reappearing with another personality, it's just hell' (a mother about her son).

Hostility is almost never apparent unless there are high levels of criticism, and is very rarely needed to define high EE relatives on its own. Ratings of hostility tend to mean that relationships between carers and patients are almost at breaking point. It may require considerable therapeutic skill to improve them, and alternatives such as patients and relatives living apart should be seriously considered.

Criticism and Feedback

We have emphasized the distinction between the lay and the technical concepts of criticism. We must also underline the difference between relatives' criticism as we have described it and the provision of feedback — 'constructive criticism' in common parlance. Avoiding the negative style of relating reflected by critical comments does not mean that relatives cannot talk frankly with patients about things they find upsetting. Indeed, relatives need to be very clear about such things, as we discuss in detail on p. 131.

The therapist must be instrumental in encouraging new styles of providing feedback. Patients are unable to meet the requirements of relatives when expressed in such negatively loaded terms — they back off. Each point of view is rather easily lost in this negative spiral and, in the end, nobody listens to anyone any more. Communication is restricted and relatives feel under restraint.

Sometimes, however, it is the relatives who back off, and no limits are set to the patients' actions — no feedback is provided at all, and unacceptable behaviour continues or worsens. This can be a very difficult and dangerous scenario that requires the provision of a clear structure from therapists. Finally the third ineffective solution to the problem of giving feedback is to attempt to outshout the patient. It can be imagined how unsuccessful this is; it is unlikely to meet anyone's needs, particularly if they happen to suffer from a mental illness.

The Role of Education in Reducing Criticism

Changing critical attitudes and behaviour requires a prolonged transfer of information. The initial provision of factual material as embodied in the educational elements of the research intervention packages described on pp. 59–65 is a small part of this process. The real education of relatives is very subtle and prolonged — it is not after all about passing an examination — and involves a radical transformation of attitudes and emotional reactions through experiences that the therapist must seek to shape.

In order to set about changing these attitudes, and to help direct and defuse the anger and resentment underlying them, the essential first step is to offer the alternative interpretation that patients are ill. This implies they are not deliberately trying to upset or frustrate carers, but that their difficult behaviour arises because they are not always in control of their frightening and worrying preoccupations and may no longer be totally in touch with reality.

The purpose of offering information to relatives may appear blindingly obvious: an attempt to help them understand and then cope with what is happening to the patient and themselves. However, it is lent added point by findings that highly critical relatives are mainly unaware of the likely effects of mental illness (Vaughn and Leff, 1976a; Gantt et al., 1989).

This means that in very critical families it is possible to begin the process of defusing resentment by providing relatives with an alternative explanation. This is particularly the case for the negative symptoms, which are very difficult to understand, common in the long-term group, and, in contrast to the positive symptoms, unlikely to respond well to medication.

A major theme in the history of social psychiatry has been the application of labelling theory (Goffman, 1961; Scheff, 1966). While it is clear that the process of labelling sometimes has untoward effects on the behaviour of professional staff, leading to an inflexible response towards patients, we would argue that it also has benefits. This is particularly so where the provision of a label to the relatives of people with persistent disabilities allows them to change their attributions of the other person's behaviour in a way that improves the relationship. This viewpoint implies an acceptance that the concept of schizophrenia has elements that are not social (that it is a disease, if you like). We ourselves have no difficulty over this.

Clearly the mere provision of a label without amplification risks all the adverse consequences set out by the anti-labelling polemicists. For it to be constructive, it must therefore be accompanied by a clear and detailed description of its implications, in so far as they are known.

This emphasizes the value of offering education to carers. It involves giving them new, and often unwelcome information about what the problems consist of, and thus how the carer can begin to cope differently with the worries.

Understanding and Tolerating Symptoms

As professionals we have been trained to distinguish symptoms from ordinary behaviour. Relatives have to make this distinction for themselves, so it is not surprising that they often fail to do so and as a result react unhelpfully. Socially embarrassing behaviour and negative symptoms are most difficult for relatives to deal with, but at least the former are easy to see as the effect of mental illness. They are also less persistent and often lead to active intervention on the part of staff. Researchers are currently investigating the value of training relatives and patients to spot the re-emergence of active symptoms at an early stage, so that prompt action can be taken to preempt a full blown relapse.

Negative symptoms as we have stressed repeatedly are more common and persistent, and more difficult to deal with. Features like lack of interest, lack of motivation, lack of energy, and social withdrawal are those that cause most trouble to experienced carers (Creer and Wing, 1975). Apathy and inactivity provokes only an incomprehending frustration in the onlooker. Relatives often respond with misplaced enthusiasm to the slightest sign of interest in anything. One of our patients suddenly expressed an interest in fishing to his father, who immediately rushed out and purchased an expensive set of fishing tackle. It was never used. On another occasion, the son mentioned an interest in some piece of music and his father again impetuously bought a complete stereo music system, also unused. These actions are a clear indication of the desperation that is sometime felt by loving parents who fail to understand the nature of the condition their children suffer from. The effect is an understandable but unfortunate increase in the parents' sense of frustration and enragement.

In such circumstances, it is crucial for the therapist to help the relatives to see that apathy has to be dealt with in more mundane and persistent ways, with much lower expectations. Relatively esoteric activities are rarely the answer. It is much more to the point to encourage the patient to rise from bed a little earlier, to do a little more in the way of self-care, to take part just a little more often in family activities. The aim is to get the patient back into any sort of routine, be it ever so commonplace. This involves concentration on simple things, perhaps the repetition of some small task, just to get the patient back into a rhythm. This serves as the groundwork for slightly more demanding things later on.

The establishment of a modest programme for progress often requires the therapist to persuade relatives to hold off, as part of inculcating a proper pace and perspective. They need to alter their expectations of what patients may go back to. One of our patients was a fine cricket player: after his illness, it was not possible for him to take this up actively again, particularly as his social withdrawal would have made it too difficult for him to take part in a team game in an effective way. However, he did get back to watching it on television; he enjoyed this, and it was possible to use his readiness to talk about the game to encourage social interaction. Another patient with an interest in astronomy was incapable of engaging in observing directly, yet could be encouraged to buy astronomy magazines and read the less technical and more interesting articles with mild enthusiasm.

Understanding Medication

An equally important reason for explaining the negative symptoms is the need to defuse arguments about drug treatment.

These can take up an inordinate amount of time and energy, but may be short-circuited if carers and patients are helped to understand the function of medication.

Unless provided with information to the contrary, most carers and many patients believe that the negative symptoms, which tend to become more salient as acute symptoms subside, are the direct result of the major tranquillizers given to reduce the latter. Relatives may well have been told about the possibility of side effects, and in today's climate they are very likely to be familiar with the idea. There are real problems in any case because there is an overlap between negative symptoms and the side effects of major tranquillizers, and professionals themselves may be in doubt in the individual case. It is therefore a complex and grey area.

Therapists probably require to be quite explicit about this, saying that there is clearly a possibility of overlap, but that negative symptoms do exist over and above the effects of medication and are the more likely reason for the patients' behaviour. After all, behavioural deficits were frequent in patients with schizophrenia long before effective medication was available. In general, it should be explained that the existence of negative symptoms is a bad argument for discontinuing medication.

It is important to deal clearly with issues about medication, because therapists may otherwise find that relatives and patients gang up on them in an unproductive way. Relatives plainly know very little about medication and its effects (eg. Gantt et al., 1989). If anyone has been informed, it is most likely to have been the patient, who was probably not in a wholly receptive state of mind at the time. It is possible that information about medication will have to be provided more than once, and even then relatives still may not believe what the therapist says. Their views may be coloured by previous misconceptions, and these may be hard to shift. A common one is the confusion between major and minor tranquillizers, such that prevalent and valid worries about the addictiveness of minor tranquillizers may be applied inappropriately to the major group. There is in any case current concern about the value of pharmacological treatment in general, deriving variously from the environmental movement, holistic medicine and principles of self-help. This means that the therapist must be prepared to engage in a clear discussion with patients and relatives about where the balance of advantage to the patient lies in the individual case. The therapist should make the effort to unpack the situation. In the process, both patients and relatives must be given space to voice their concerns.

It may be possible for patients to agree that even though they do not like medication, taking it is better than the prospect of relapse. Sometimes alternative strategies may be feasible. So for example it may be possible to decrease the frequency of oral medication, either by reducing the overall dose, or by redistributing it. On other occasions, patients may find long-acting injections a preferable alternative. This is a good example of a situation in which flexibility on the therapist's part brings dividends.

Carers tend to assume that, once the patient is 'better', medication is no longer necessary. This may in any case be exactly how patients feel, and so they join with carers in confronting staff with the easy target of 'he doesn't need this medication'. The concept of prophylaxis is a hard one to communicate.

Helping carers and patients (and sometimes staff) to understand that psychotic illnesses have both positive and negative symptoms, and that the effects of medication are predominantly on the reduction and continued suppression of the former, may take some time, but it is usually important to concentrate on it as a first step. Patients may well feel that they are made worse on medication, and fail to notice any benefits. The decision to prescribe medication on a long-term basis is a serious one that requires families to understand the implications. If they agree, they risk side effects, but the hoped for reward is the suppression of acute symptoms; if they disagree they risk disruptive relapses and crises. Professionals who fail to inform families of the rationale for long-term medication are unlikely to be able to enlist their support in encouraging the patients' compliance. Nor will they be able to do so if the professionals' own grounds for advising medication are poorly thought out.

Thus the object of all this explanation is to separate out the behaviour caused by the effects of illness, the effects of medication and the patient's own reaction. The object is not necessarily achieved of course. The mother of a 45 year old man, who had stayed in bed most of the time until we managed to persuade him to the day centre, continued to maintain that he was 'lazy'. While she listened to our explanations, and could eventually see that her son did have difficulties in achieving things — getting up, managing to come to the workshop despite feeling tired — and that the medication was not the only reason he was like this, she has never really agreed with us that he had been ill. She still thinks he could do more to help himself. To some extent she is probably right, but it would be better if we could get her to help him with his motivation, rather than to criticize him for not having any.

Changing Expectations

Once relatives have achieved some understanding of why patients are behaving in difficult or bizarre ways, the next stage is to help them change their expectations so that they may choose realistic and achievable objectives. Expecting patients to return to 'normal' or to 'go back to work' after many years of illness is usually a recipe for disappointment: at the very least, it will take a very long time. Nevertheless carers often have expectations like this — they may assume that patients' problems will disappear, that a severe psychotic illness is merely a passing phase. Such opinions are almost bound to result in a prolonged and unproductive sense of frustration. In turn, this engenders the view that patients are not trying, and can add to the feelings of failure, loss of confidence and depression so common among patients in the recovery phase of a severe psychotic illness.

In order for staff members, carers and patients to achieve change, it is necessary for aims to be pitched at the correct level. Successes must be seen against the yardstick of the possible: 'she hardly ever bothers to go to that day centre' and 'she hardly ever gets there, but its such an effort I'm pleased when she does' are references to the same activity. However the more positive inter-pretation enables carer and patient to feel that change might after all be possible, and allows an incipient optimism about efforts to help. The first description disregards the effort, and denigrates its importance. It thus becomes a self-fulfilling belief in the impossibility of change.

Where families themselves are too immersed in a problem to be able to see minor changes, staff have a particular role, as they are much better placed to resolve issues into small components that can then be the focus of attempted modification. It is also important of course for staff to do this for each other: to specify small goals that are achievable and to mark when they occur. Small gains are important, and must be made to seem so to all concerned: working for a couple of hours in a workshop three afternoons a week may be a giant leap for a patient who has been sitting at home doing almost nothing for the previous six months.

Perspective

It is very easy for relatives of patients with longstanding illness to say nothing ever changes. Staff often say it too: 'I remember Fred when he was in the long stay ward — he's exactly the same now as he was then' — even though Fred may now be living in a much less institutionalized setting. It is sometimes much easier to live with the resignation and pessimism of perceived immutability, than to examine a situation in detail and endure the risk involved in agreeing that there might have been a small improvement. In order to see changes, it is often useful to evaluate the patient's status over a long perspective. This may reveal change that has been extremely gradual, subject to reversals, and limited to a few areas. For instance, the fact that Fred is no longer particularly violent, manages with much less supervision (indeed none at night), and is no longer a particular worry to staff, can be presented as quite a large change for someone with as many disabilities as he has. If this is pointed out to staff members and carers alike, it may come as a revelation. Persuading and assisting carers to look back over, say, a year, may often enable small changes to be seen more distinctly. Even if there have been bad patches, they may have been shorter or less frequent than in the past. Recovery may be a little quicker, remission a little more prolonged. These gains may sound trivial, but enabling carers and staff to take a longer view is usually valuable, given that even maintaining the status quo might be a considerable achievement with some of the more fragile patients. If there is a deterioration, looking back at the pattern of previous relapses or crises may help reassure relatives or staff that the episode is very similar and therefore likely to respond to treatment, or to be contained more effectively because it was noticed early.

As helping carers to see progress, even when it is very slow, and to appreciate changes in the quality of a very disabled life is a means of maintaining their hope, it also sustains their interest in patients, and their commitment to caring for them.

A final consequence of sharing information, providing understanding and promoting tolerance, realistic expectations and a true perspective of the time scale of change is that it can help staff, relatives and patients work together rather than against each other. Replacing mutual recrimination with an open sharing of problems, information, and the difficulties of the tasks signifies the beginning of useful engagement in the process of long-term care. Because of the risk of reversals and consequent discouragement, supportive relationships between all sides of the triangle — patient, carer and staff — are crucial for enabling all concerned to weather problems constructively. If such relationships cannot be fostered, the slightest whiff of adversity may result in an adversarial and destructive confrontation.

The Role of Problem Solving

Principles and strategies of problem solving are discussed in detail in Chapter 8. However, there are specific issues relevant to its application in interventions with critical relatives. It is crucial to encourage relatives to adopt different styles of coping and different approaches to problems. There is much better chance of success and therefore of self-reinforcement if relatives will try something different.

However, there is a real problem for therapists in this. Although they must encourage relatives to search for alternative ways for them to manage their situation, they must avoid the suggestion that relatives were previously doing things wrong. If relatives perceive the therapists' encouragement as denigrating their previous efforts, they will not commit themselves to the need for change. It is therefore useful for therapists to point out to relatives what was good in their previous attempts — this is not too difficult, as most such attempts have their good aspects even when they fail.

Involving critical relatives in problem solving allows therapists to help them to increase their consistency and their repertoire, and to pitch their efforts at the right level, and thus to break out of seemingly intractable situations.

One family we deal with consists of a mother and two sons living in rather cramped accommodation. One son has a lot of physical symptoms and is under a variety of clinics. Our patient is the other son who typically reverses day and night — he sleeps all day and gets up at night to watch the video. This sleep pattern has at times enraged the other two family members who are woken up at night. It has been very difficult to help the family reorganize their routine, and the process is still continuing.

We have helped the family redefine the problem as one of adult autonomy. Peter does have the right to organize his life without the others interfering, but he now also recognizes that his getting up at night is disturbing. With this as a basis, a new schedule was agreed such that Peter would try to watch TV in the day, and get his sleep pattern back into a more ordinary routine. It also emerged that he is able to go shopping for the family, and even though this is often in the evenings, his relatives recognize it as a helpful contribution on his part. Once the new schedule was agreed, Peter had difficulties in sticking to it; moreover any backsliding led to disproportionate complaints from his relatives. However, he has increased his general day time activities and often manages to go to bed by 10 pm, although we are still trying to help his mother and brother see this behaviour as encouraging. For the moment, we as staff have taken on the role of being positive to Peter about his progress in the hope his relatives can respond to this example. This not only enables the family to consider a different way of interacting, but enhances Peter's motivation to maintain new behaviour patterns, until his family are more able to do this themselves.

This example exhibits both the policy and some of the difficulties of using a structured approach to problems in order to modify criticism. Here the family situation demanded (and still demands) stalwart persistence and dedication from the staff involved.

6·*Overinvolvement*

'The going was really hard, I was just about at breaking point'. (A father speaking of his daughter).

Characteristics of Overinvolvement

Overinvolvement is a complicated attribute with several components. These include overprotectiveness and a tendency towards self sacrifice. Relatives displaying overinvolvement often appear somewhat dramatic in recounting their situation, which they may do in an excessive degree of detail. It appears as though they are obsessively interested in routine details of their circumstances.

Most people are upset when their relatives have to be admitted to hospital. Identifying overinvolvement within this upset means that we are attempting to recognize the extreme of what is a continuum of behaviour. It is not merely a matter of evaluating anxiety in the face of admission, but also the notable impact it is having on the relative — 'It felt like death', 'I lost two stone in weight', 'I had to follow him everywhere around the house'.

The last phrase from these examples emphasizes the nature of reactions characterizing overinvolvement — the need to supervise, to control in order to preempt bad things happening. At difficult times, this is a common way of expressing care. The problem with overinvolvement is that this style of caring is carried over into situations where it ceases to be appropriate; such relatives appearing unable to modify their behaviour in response to changing circumstances.

In some respects, the behaviour is a bit like treating patients as children. Relatives perceive (accurately) that patients are less able to cope with aspects of their lives. In consequence, they take over some of the patients' functions as they would do with a child. The patients, however, are not in fact children, there is always a sense in which this is inappropriate, and relatives are unable to draw the line clearly. This has similarities with Minuchin's concept of enmeshment (1974) — the situation in which people are unable to separate appropriately what their roles and functions are and should be.

Overinvolvement is usually more typical of the parents of patients than spouses or cohabitees, presumably because it is a reversion to a pattern of behaviour well-learned during the patients' childhood years. However, it appears to be within the repertoire of a minority of spouses and of other carers as well.

A common consequence of overinvolvement is intrusiveness. Relatives are unable to leave patients alone and may go to extremes, for example continually following them around the house. If patients try to retreat to their bedroom, the relatives go too. Again, this is not necessarily a mistake; after all staff may place patients under constant supervision at times of crisis. However, it becomes so when it is done incessantly, and when the acute stage is resolved.

The central issue is of *independence*, deciding how much independence it is appropriate to allow patients. This is particularly difficult in longstanding illness, because the relatives perceive accurately that patients are deficient in a variety of skills. They may be poor managers of money, or they may be open to exploitation by others, both financially and sexually. They may have real problems in taking decisions for themselves or in taking responsibility for themselves generally.

Given that problems are real, relatives need judgement over where to draw the line between what is reasonable and what is not. This can be particularly difficult where the patients' difficulties are extreme and longstanding. Indeed, in these circumstances, staff members themselves have parallel problems, and frequently render the patient more dependent than is actually necessary. Clearly what is difficult for staff, who have the advantage of a degree of detachment, must be doubly so for enmeshed relatives.

Overinvolvement is often associated with unrealistic perceptions of the patient, and indeed the persistence of this type of behaviour may derive at least partly from this distorted view. The relatives are unable to see patients as they currently are, they are very unclear about their current deficits and assets. They are however aware that things are not as they should be, and often hark back to the past and to how patients used to be — 'he was such a beautiful child', 'he was always so good at school'

— in a way that both expresses puzzlement and avoids any realistic contemplation of the problems and difficulties that will now be, perhaps to a considerable degree, an inevitable accompaniment of the patients' lives. In extreme cases, relatives will shower nothing but praise on patients, in a manner that looks positive but is actually a denial and an obstruction to any possibility of progress: 'He's wonderful; there are never any problems'. This behaviour prevents things being changed for the better, and is often seen as a slight by patients, who know that things are far from wonderful but feel stymied by the massive obstructiveness created by this false and fulsome praise. It denies the reality of their difficulties and blocks the pathways to help and change.

In terms of helping patients and their relatives, the problem with overinvolvement is that it rigidifies their relationship in a way that does not take account of the actual nature of the difficulties they face. Although the issue does concern patients making their own decisions and taking responsibility for their lives, patients after all are not children, and any resemblances in behaviour are superficial. Nevertheless, the fear of relatives concerns decisions that might go wrong (as they do sometimes for all of us), and as a result they attempt to eliminate the possibility of bad consequences and to control situations by taking over all decisions from the patients. The outcome of this is to 'deskill' and 'derole' patients, and to prevent the acquisition of new skills and repertoires.

By some (not all) patients, this is seen as intrusive and suffocating. The result may be destructive and painful arguments over a whole string of what look like minor matters. For instance, there may be arguments about whether patients should go out for a walk alone. Relatives resist this because of a fear of the consequences of even this apparently straightforward activity. In other cases, relatives and patients may not even be able to discuss an issue like this: argument is out of scope within the culture of the family.

Overinvolvement is a complex set of behaviours, considerably more so than criticism, which is a relatively simple response comprised of not liking and not understanding some aspect of the patient's behaviour. Overinvolvement, in contrast, is compounded of a whole range of possible emotional responses — guilt, fear, anxiety, grief, denial, protectiveness. It somehow seems to have far greater reverberations than criticism for the nature of the relationship. This is probably reflected in the fact that interventions with relatives have tended to have greater success in shifting criticism than overinvolvement (e.g. Leff et al., 1982).

Vulnerability

The sticking point for overinvolved relatives is that they know for a fact that patients are vulnerable. Their attempts to control the patients' environment, although carrying long-term disadvantages, has a considerable basis in rationality. Protectiveness is both reasonable and to be appreciated in those caring for people with longstanding mental illness. After all their disabilities may well never disappear. Even when patients are managing well, they may have lost skills in numerous aspects of everyday living. They may lack competence in budgetting, and they may be particularly poor at dealing with relationships because of a loss of interest and of the required high level emotional skills. They are often incapable of handling unexpected situations.

As a result of these disabilities, they are particularly open to financial or sexual exploitation. Relatives may worry that patients are vulnerable even when they go for a walk — because they may be unalert, preoccupied or unskilled, they may be particularly open to attack or robbery, especially in an inner city area like ours. Although the patients' sexuality can be virtually a taboo subject, many relatives are very worried about the dangers of sexual relationships for patients — the possibility of pregnancy, the choosing of inappropriate partners, the risk of sexual exploitation or merely of stormy relationships.

Not every long-term patient has these problems. However, many do, and carers may want to restrict their freedom to wander or to handle money. This is particularly so when patients first became ill in adolescence. They may then never have acquired skills in the first place, and their relatives will have had no experience of dealing with them as autonomous adults.

Protectiveness therefore has good grounds. Carried to extremes, however, it limits the patients' development. Risks occasionally have to be taken in the name of progress, but relatives with the habit of vigilance may feel progress is not worth any risk. It is true that patients seem infinitely susceptible to stress, but stresses are finally unavoidable, and the relatives' attempts to anticipate every eventuality may result in a restrictive overprotectiveness that needs to be modified. In other cases, drawing the line between a wise and caring protectiveness and a counterproductive excess is not so easy: it involves issues like quality of life, and there may be no definitive answer. It requires fine judgement on the part of the professional through consultation with patients and carers.

When the relatives' fears are partly grounded in reality, it can be very difficult to engender changes in the family system that will permit greater separation and independence. Change will usually be a slow process, as it can be very difficult to reassure relatives sufficiently so they will allow it. It may indeed be necessary to accept that goals will have to be limited. Occasionally, the psychiatric team may have to wait until the relative dies before full plans for encouraging independence in the patient can be implemented. In the meantime, an undesirable level of interdependence will persist between relative and patient, and the lives of both will be less full than they might be. When the team's best efforts at persuasion fail, it is better to acknowledge it and live with it — it is important then to accept more limited aims with a good grace. These will certainly include providing support where necessary and maintaining contact with the family.

Parental Overinvolvement and the Problems of Sexuality

The parents of mentally ill daughters may be particularly worried by the possibility of promiscuous behaviour. This fear is sometimes based on fantasy but may not be. A much loved child, who may have been shy before the illness began, seems to lose discrimination and chooses as sexual partners people who would previously have been considered as unlikely or unsuitable in some way. Sometimes relatives feel particularly concerned because patients appear vulnerable to sexual advances, and they worry that outsiders could be taking advantage. This can be a very upsetting problem: the normal tendency to accept the desire of adults for independence and sexual freedom conflicts with their wish to protect a loved child from sexual abuse or hurt. For adult patients, there is rarely any way to enforce sexual rules. Even though carers dislike it, they may have to accept a certain amount of independence and sexual freedom. Relatives should be encouraged with delicacy and tact, to *support* patients through these relationships. They should try to show that they still care, despite patients acting in ways they would not choose them to. Help with *contraception* is usually relevant and important, and relatives may be those best able to suggest and organize this.

Parents find it particularly difficult to accept this side of a patient's adult life. The parents of one woman in her early thirties were distressed by her going off for several nights with an unknown man, after which she had returned home dishevelled and uncommunicative. They never did hear the full details of this episode. Thereafter they tended to be rather protective of her, and discouraged male friends from phoning or calling round. In this family, the patient was herself not worried by her lack of a boyfriend, and she did not disagree with her parents' attitude. It can be much more difficult if this becomes an area of dispute in the family, and has to be sorted out in some way that respects the patient's adult needs.

Many patients seek sexual outlets when they are relatively well, but even this may be very difficult for their relatives to contemplate, particularly if the patient is female and lives at home. Problems arise over privacy and the practicalities of conducting a relationship under these circumstances. Relatives may find the chosen sexual partner wholly unacceptable — after all patients often have a limited range of contacts from which to choose. Indeed, 10% of our patients are living with each other. It may be particularly difficult for relatives to accept that patients' partners may have their own disabilities.

In cases of mania, promiscuity may only be apparent for some of the time. It may then be an early sign of relapse. If this is pointed out to carers, they can be primed to enlist the team's help at an early stage.

Pregnancy is unlikely if effective contraception is provided; however, we have come across patients who want a sexual relationship but refuse to contemplate contraception. In these circumstances, one must make the potential consequences very clear to them: patients with long-term illness often lose custody of their children. This must be done not in the manner of a threat, but through an open and realistic discussion.

In the remainder of this chapter, we discuss specific problems for professional staff in helping overinvolved relatives.

The Role of Education in Reducing Overinvolvement

Conveying basic information about the patients' condition and situation is always difficult when relatives are feeling worried and anxious, and this response is universal in overinvolved relatives, particularly at times of crisis. The danger of education is that it may reinforce anxiety in the overinvolved by emphasizing the fact of illness. Relatives may respond to this information with 'well, I'd better look after him then', and end up by taking over yet more roles and responsibilities.

It is therefore crucial to emphasize to such relatives that it can be caring to let patients become independent, even within reason to allow them to make mistakes, provided they are at least their own mistakes. The changes in the abilities of patients as their more acute symptoms abate should also be stressed, suggesting that as they improve, they should be encouraged to make at least some of their own decisions and choices, and to accept an increasing responsibility for their own well being and self-care. By emphasizing the variation in the course of the disorder, it may be possible to get relatives to moderate, at least to some extent, the rigidity of their expectations and their behaviour.

Discussing the Worst Outcome

A good way to start with overinvolved relatives is to discuss their fears of the worst foreseeable outcome to particular situations. The reason for overinvolvement and the consequent taking over of responsibilities is often that the relatives have fantasies about a very bad outcome indeed if they do not take over. Sometimes something awful has indeed happened in the past — we know of a patient who did set the kitchen on fire in the process of making a cup of tea. To some extent therefore the fantasies may be grounded in actuality, but they are rarely totally realistic. Relatives will restrict patients (and themselves in a different sense) 'just in case', just to block the possibility of something going wrong. Patients may never be left alone, never allowed to make tea, never permitted to do the shopping or to have their own money.

In such circumstances, it is often a good strategy to specify the worst fear, and to discuss what can be done if it comes to pass. The therapist should then discuss the relatives' fantasies in the context of what really does happen, to unpack how realistic the worst fears actually are. For instance, parents may worry that their daughter might be robbed or made pregnant. Clearly these things do happen, but the therapist must evaluate how realistic these fears are in the individual case. Are they mere fantasy or might they reflect a real possibility? If the latter, how can it be minimized?

It usually needs quite detailed discussion to establish what is dangerous and what connotes an acceptable degree of risk. It may turn out, for instance, that relatives were wrong in thinking patients were seeking a sexual relationship when they were only asking for friendship and someone to talk to. It is usually possible to sort out a compromise. For example, parents may be worried about a daughter spending evenings with her boyfriend away from home, but it may transpire that she would find it equally acceptable to spend time with him during the day. Once the process of negotiation has begun, it may not be difficult to see alternatives that serve the needs of everyone concerned.

Attention should then be turned to considering what is reasonable in guarding against situations for which the fears have some basis in fact. Ideally, a specific fear should be related to a specific solution, so, if fire is a genuine hazard, it might be reasonable to negotiate with patients that they do not have matches in their possession. This focus on practical solutions to individual problems can initiate the break up of a protectiveness that has become too overinclusive.

In this context, it can be very reassuring for relatives to attend a group where they can meet other relatives in similar situations and learn that the fears they are concerned about are in fact very common.

Occasionally, despite all their efforts, relatives and staff may still be obliged to see patients fail at something — to spend all their money or to have an unplanned baby. Such happenings are quite tragic, but it may yet be possible for patients to learn something from the experience and even come to terms with what they can realistically manage for themselves. Insight may gradually emerge as a result, though it is a hard way to learn.

Permissions

One important function of staff who support relatives is to give them 'permission' to have a life of their own, separate from the patient. This is essential for both relative and patient, especially when the former shows overinvolvement. The staff member must get it across to relatives that it is all right for them to do things by and for themselves, as well as being care-givers. Many relatives have not thought this through, and feel irrationally that they are 'not allowed' to have any good times. 'Even if I went out, I'd feel bad about leaving him at home, I'd feel guilty about him sitting there alone'.

It is difficult to erode such feelings, but an essential approach is to promote small separations as *beneficial for the patient* — indeed they are the antithesis of self sacrifice with its deskilling effects. Obviously this must be done in a manner that avoids adding to relatives' guilt. It may be helpful to emphasize what is true, that relatives may find the stress of 24-hour care too much to bear, and that this may lead to a diminished efficiency and even to mental health problems of their own. These will in turn reduce their ability to provide the very care they are committed to. In other words, they will be better carers for allowing themselves time off. It is important for the wellbeing of patients to get relatives to a position where they feel able to acknowledge that they have needs of their own.

Another method for leading older relatives to accept support in the difficult role of carer is to discuss what will happen when they die. This is a good way of getting them to see the downside of overprovision of care. Many elderly relatives are already worried about this issue, and so it is productive for staff members to address this worry and the problem of overinvolvement simultaneously. Under the circumstances it may be fairly easy to persuade relatives of the disadvantages of making themselves irreplaceable. It can be put to them that it is important to encourage patients towards greater independence while they are still in a position to promote it. In this way, they can be helped to accept the necessity for letting go to an extent, and to allow patients a greater role in decision making.

Focusing on specific targets

Clearly, it is insufficient merely to suggest to relatives and patients that they should spend more time apart. The therapist must be more specific. It may be reasonable to suggest an hour apart on a particular day, or that relatives should have an evening out (separations at weekends are usually less feasible). A useful approach is to try and get relatives to attend for an appointment *without* the patient. Relatives should then be encouraged to evaluate the consequences, for example, that the house and the patient are actually still OK when they return. In other words, the feared worst outcome is not confirmed.

Most patients actually engage in embarrassing, destructive or dangerous behaviour fairly rarely, and persuading relatives to acknowledge this can be a useful first stage for therapists to build on.

Dealing with the worry is often more difficult than setting the task. However, there may sometimes be problems initially in making the task small enough — for instance, choosing a form of separation inconsequential enough to be feasible.

Attempts at increasing patients' independence must be framed within a knowledge of their residual disabilities. This may mean focusing on relatively trifling aspects of self-care (which may not be trifling to patient or relative). It may be possible to get patients to contribute to minor household tasks, or to be more responsible for self-care — taking baths more often, looking after their room.

Relatives often take on an enormous amount of physical care of patients, some of which may be appropriate, some not. This may include, for instance, bathing them. One way of diluting this degree of physical care is for staff members to share some of the responsibility. It is sometimes possible to arrange for patients to bathe at a day centre. This can in any case be a way of encouraging attendance. Moreover, staff may be able to take on this task in a way which allows patients more responsibility — so they may escort them to the bath, but decline to wash them physically, although relatives may actually be doing this.

In this instance, relatives are doing something which may be quite appropriate, although the manner of doing it may not be the best possible. By having staff members take over part of the responsibility it is possible to avoid suggesting the behaviour is inappropriate, while preventing it at least some of the time. As staff are likely to be more flexible in the degree of assistance offered, an increased independence can thus be fostered, and this in turn can be used to chip away at the relatives' overconcern.

This example emphasizes the fundamental problem of the level of functioning that should be aimed at. The experience of illness may change patients' own targets of self-care, social activity, and so on. Good management must therefore often be about reaching an adult compromise, but this implies using the normal adult population as a benchmark rather than the level of functioning to be expected of a child.

Limit Setting

The practicalities of limit setting are dealt with in the following chapters, but the issue is of particular relevance to overinvolved relatives. They typically find it very difficult to set appropriate and consistent limits, and as a result are often landed with behaviour that they feel is unacceptable. They often become furious as a result, but hide these feelings. This is again reminiscent of a particular style of childcare, although there may be an added factor of fear as patients are adult and may retaliate. The result may be that relatives let patients do what they like, and make no demands upon them, even at some cost to themselves. Some get angry, others merely exhausted.

Because they do not think of patients as adult, relatives may find it hard to get them to take responsibility. The consequence is often both overinvolvement *and* criticism, a very complicated emotion: 'I love him, I hate him'. The role of the therapist must be to help both sides behave in an adult way, to have reasonable and realistic expectations of each other. This involves helping relatives to set limits without resorting to argument or violence, which are common consequences when the situation has been allowed to fester over a long period. The essential procedure is to assist in the negotiation of mutually agreed limits. Relatives then need to be firm in a clear way rather than an angry one.

It is very hard for overinvolved relatives to get the balance right over setting limits, and it is a key area in which staff members should provide support. Gradually patients should be encouraged to take on more tasks, with a consequent shaping of skills leading to greater independence. This includes both doing more around the house and doing more socially.

Structure

Often patients living with overinvolved relatives become very deskilled, partly as a result of the process of illness, partly as a result of disuse inadvertently encouraged by the relative. A way round this is through the provision of structure. The clinical team can do this by encouraging patients to use facilities outside the home, such as day centres, day hospitals, sheltered work. The mere obligation to get up and get out will provide some structure to the patients' day and emphasize that activity even at a low level of competence is of some value. Being obliged to attend an outside facility means that patients are exposed to people who treat them in a more adult way, and in a different setting. It thus opens the door to a training or a reemergence of skills, even though the level of functioning required at first may initially seem to be trivial.

The problem for many patients enmeshed with overinvolved relatives is that they may never engage in *any* outside activity. This situation and the relationship with the relative may be quite comfortable, and this makes separation even more difficult to achieve, and likely to require a long time.

In some cases, the first feasible step may be to get relatives out of the house, for part-time work, adult education classes, and so on. Once this has been achieved, it may then also be possible to persuade patients to do something outside the home, providing more opportunities for the 'adult' to emerge.

Patients who become ill in adolescence may indeed never have achieved much adult independence; schizophrenia can block the path very effectively, freezing skills at their pre-illness level. This may result in the need to start at very low levels of expectation even in someone who is 30 or 40 years old. Starting at a low point demands easy targets and limited expectations. It is important that this should be clear to all concerned.

Special Problems

A difficult situation exists where one relative is overinvolved, and another critical. This is not infrequent where patients still live with parents, and can lead to endless marital disagreement, tensions and arguments. It gives great scope for patients to play one parent off against the other, a process that staff members may become involved in to the detriment of consistent and effective management.

In such a case, the parents will differ in their approach to virtually every problem. They may be more concerned to score points off each other than to arrive at a genuinely helpful solution.

Management under these circumstances is difficult. It requires the therapist to promote two changes at the same time. This involves educating the critical relative, providing a different model of response, and attempting to get them to reattribute the patient's behaviour in a manner that is less destructive, while persuading the overinvolved relative that being caring can mean allowing the patient space. Attempts should be made to get the relatives to be consistent over one selected problem area. This is difficult to effect, but serves as a model for cooperative behaviour in other departments. The process requires fine judgement on the therapist's part, between damping down the overinvolvement and enhancing the quality of caring in the critical relative.

It may be tempting to try and improve the marital relationship itself. However, realism is required here. Sometimes, the best that can be managed is for the relatives to work together on the problems faced by and created by the patient.

One way or another, relatives of this pattern are wrapped up in the patients and their difficulties — this may be the only thing keeping them together in the same house, and they may not be motivated to improve their marriage. Such circumstances demand very careful thought: probing too deeply into matters the relatives may want to be left unexamined may kill the opportunity for cooperation in areas where it is possible. Spouses do not have to like each other very much, provided they both care what happens to their mentally ill offspring, and are able to cooperate at least over this.

As suggested above, it is not uncommon for criticism and overinvolvement to coexist in a carer. Again, this needs careful handling by the therapist to increase relatives' understanding and tolerance at the same time as suggesting that they might back off a little. Difficulties often arise over setting limits, which may be chosen inappropriately. The way around difficulties with limits is usually to involve patients in the process of deciding what they should be, and this is a strong argument for dealing with relatives combining criticism with overinvolvement in a family setting rather than through relatives' groups. The aim is then to replace wild oscillations in the relatives' behaviour with consistency. Critical overinvolved relatives frequently meet suggestions of possible ways of handling specific problems with 'Oh, I've tried that'. This often turns out to be true, but they may have only adopted the strategy suggested on a single occasion, and sometimes not an auspicious one at that. They therefore need to be led to a more persistent application of potential solutions.

The difficulty of persuading relatives into new strategies is that they worry it will fail. The status quo may be bad, but at least it is familiar and thus just within the bounds of the endurable. The therapist therefore requires to be reassuring about any proposed changes. An impression must be created that the therapist will hold the situation steady, and 'catch' the family if it goes wrong. This means persuading the relative and the patient to trust staff, to feel that they can be reached in a crisis, that they do not necessarily have to go back through the family doctor, that they are not going to be let down. As this may be completely counter to their previous experience with service-providers, it may not be easy to gain trust in this way.

7·Coping with Emotions

One of the most noticeable aspects of this kind of work is an emotional burden that spares none of those involved. Carers typically experience a whole range of emotional responses from shock, grief, guilt and worries about the vulnerability of patients to anger, rejection, stigma, isolation, fear of the future and despair.

Staff members feel similar emotions at times, although they are less likely to experience stigma or isolation. They are also likely to feel impotent, helpless and frustrated, particularly with patients who do not change unless for the worse.

The emotions of patients likewise range from loss of confidence, poor self esteem, and feelings of worthlessness and rejection from stigmatization and marginalization, to depression and despair. Hopelessness is often compounded by the grinding poverty of living only on state benefits and in poor living conditions, particularly in the run down inner cities where many patients live.

The Responsibilities of Staff

We have good reason to doubt whether professionals are successful at tackling the emotional problems of carers. The most recent survey of the needs of carers confirms that, while practical problems were often dealt with, emotional needs were not (MacCarthy et al., 1990 (in press)). It is not possible to tell whether this was because no emotional support was offered, or because whatever is offered the relatives of the long-term group have a bottomless pit of need. The second explanation is particularly daunting, and may be one of the reasons that carers find it hard to get access to any support at all. Professional staff may worry that they will be overwhelmed by the needs of these relatives, and in consequence avoid getting too involved.

Our practical experience suggests that while the emotional needs of relatives have often been neglected, their demands can indeed *seem* unquenchable. However, one of the most important interventions that staff members can offer is to face up to these emotions, to help in containing them, and to begin the process of defusing them. It is normally not until the emotional processing has begun that relatives can accept more practical help. For instance, it is rarely possible to discuss ways whereby a patient can become more independent until the reason for the under-lying worry is tackled.

If their emotional needs are ignored, carers can become almost frantic in their search for solace. Some of the most bitter and frustrating relationships between carers and staff members seem to originate in this way. Staff not infrequently refuse to see rela-tives because they are 'too demanding'. However, this just means that others have to pick up the pieces — the police, the vicar, Salvation Army officers, the Samaritans. The response of staff members may be more subtle but no less defensive. They may not refuse to talk to relatives, but still manage to be unavailable. There are many ways of engineering this — by being patently too busy, by being called away to something more important, by referring relatives to the most junior member of staff, and so forth.

The other worry of staff members is that meeting these emo-tional needs will take too much time. Busy NHS staff cannot easily commit themselves to unlimited sessions with people who are not even designated patients. At least with practical aspects matters are reasonably clear cut — assistance is offered, accepted or otherwise, arrangements are made. Emotional support can not be so conveniently packaged, and it may take months or years to bring about demonstrable progress. This prospect does not please, and often leaves staff members feeling that it must be someone else's job!

Even if the end result of failing to deal with the relatives' emotional needs is a crisis, an emergency admission, a suicide attempt, or the patient being locked out of the house, staff find it easier to justify spending time on handling an emergency than on preventative work. This is a common position: dealing with crisis is incontravertibly a good use of staff time and effort, and normally shows fairly rapid results. Preemptive action is more mundane and can look a good deal less impressive in these days of clinical audit.

However, long-term patients do have the advantage of a history — often their problems stretch back over many years and the pattern of recurrence can be distressingly obvious. Breaking the pattern by prolonging the interval between emergency admissions, reducing relapses or sustaining less frequent, less dramatic, crises represents clear progress, although it often needs emphasis.

There is a further argument for intervening to meet emotional needs. Although the work may appear to take up a lot of time, the total commitment is unlikely to exceed that taken up in dealing with crises that would otherwise ensue. This has been confirmed in research intervention studies.

Preventive interventions do however have to be spread over several months or even years, and this implies a need for commitment and continuity. One of the most frustrating experiences of carers is the way personnel always seem to be on the move, so that each meeting may be with a new staff member. This means of course that staff are always having to go back over the history of the problem; carers and patients feel understandably and probably correctly that they are getting nowhere. It is impossible to progress with the difficult demands of emotional processing without the continuity needed to build up the relationship of trust and the familiarity with carers' problems that is an essential accompaniment. This is the starting point for meeting emotional needs. In our view it is a crucial aspect of long-term management, and should be given a proper priority.

Defusing and Containing Emotions

Two processes seem to be necessary for the successful defusion of emotions. The first is simple expression of pent-up feelings, the second the use of a variety of techniques to change carers' attitudes towards their own emotional responses.

Relatives need space to talk about upsetting things. For therapists to defuse the associated feelings, they must give time to sitting and listening. The ability of therapists to hear such things and to be accepting of them makes them more ordinary and tolerable to relatives. A fear accepted may be a fear diminished. Relatives often have very negative feelings indeed, and disconfirming their fantasies about how they may be received by other people plays a valuable part in defusing their power over the relative.

Relatives' groups have a significant role to play in this, as other members of the group will almost certainly have had similar feelings. Indeed members of staff sometimes feel very negatively about patients as well, and acknowledging this can also help to defuse the power of the relatives' emotions. Presented with evidence of the 'universality' of their situation (Yalom, 1975), relatives feel less alone and isolated. This is particularly important for the relatives of patients with longstanding illnesses, as they have often cut themselves off from friends and other social contacts because of practical difficulties, a sense of stigma, and a fear of unacceptable behaviour on the part of the patient.

Another advantage of relatives' groups in this context is that members of the group will express a whole range of experiences and feelings. Not all will be in equally difficult situations, although most will have been in the depths of despair at some time. The presence of relatives whose circumstances have improved, or who have fought their way out of a trough and have survived, can be very reassuring to those who currently feel desperate.

It is often helpful to see desperate relatives on their own, without the patient. They will then be less inhibited, and indeed they may feel unable to express negative feelings in front of the patient. They may be only too well aware that patients are sensitive and vulnerable, and be unable to handle the patients' adverse responses to criticism. Although it is not necessary in every case, many relatives of the long-term group may have to vent their feelings over an extended period. Indeed, seeing relatives alone in this way and providing a safe place for them to talk about their feelings may be the only route to family treatment of the sort described in this book. If too much is going on in the relatives' emotional world, they will be unable to listen constructively and to make the adjustments necessary for an attempt at changing things at home. They must express their feelings before anything more directly constructive can be entertained, and they have to feel safe enough to do it.

Relatives often have dire fantasies about the destructiveness and uncontrollability of their emotions, and are then terrified of the response of others should they reveal their innermost thoughts. By 'permitting' relatives to express a range of emotions both positive and negative, by being accepting of them, and by normalizing them in relation to the experiences of other relatives in a similar position, the therapist is seen to be taking control of the situation and containing the relatives' feelings. This is a particularly important function in the early stages of treatment.

It requires a combination of countenancing emotional expression with support for the relatives' situation. The therapist must respond positively to the efforts of relatives to cope, encouraging them to feel that however badly they feel about things, they have done as well as could be expected given the circumstances. Although they may be coping poorly in general, relatives have usually managed at least some issues adequately, or even well. They should be complimented for this, which can then be used as the basis for future advances.

The processes of defusing and containment may take several weeks or months, as relatives often need a period of this duration to work through the tale of how bad their situation is and how bad they feel about it. Only then can they begin to listen and advance to the next stage, that of changing their feelings. At a well chosen time, therapists should assert that it seems as though some change might be possible. If carers are attending a relatives' group, it may be feasible for the facilitator to back this up by eliciting similar timely opinions from other relatives in the group. This may lead carers to a realization that they might indeed be able to modify their situation.

Defusing Emotions by Addressing Practical Problems

At this point it is appropriate to focus on a single problem, to unpack it and to consider ways of changing it, at first be it ever so slightly. This process of focusing down is not possible when emotions are still in acute turmoil, as relatives are too busy feeling that their problems are so awful they can never be changed.

General aspects of problem solving in the families of those with longstanding mental illness are dealt with in the following chapter. However, it has a specific role in relation to the defusion and containment of emotions. In this context, the main purpose of identifying a small and potentially malleable problem is not the solution of the problem itself, but the provision of an illustrative example that can change the way relatives see their world. The problem should therefore be deliberately chosen on two grounds: because it is *not* the main focus of the relatives' worries, and because it is capable of modification. Successful change, however slight and trivial, will itself confirm the possibility of change, and of relatives taking some degree of control over their circumstances. In other words, what they do *can* have an impact.

Sometimes, however, relatives respond badly to the invitation to choose a problem for addressing in this way. Although this may reflect the relatives' inexperience in the sort of focusing required for effective problem solving, it sometimes indicates that the therapist has introduced the idea too early.

People who are very determined that their way of doing things is right are consequently resistant to change. One problem in engaging relatives in a positive initiative of the type described above is that they may see it as exposing them to criticism. If the difficulty they face really is enormous, they are not diminished by being unable to solve it — after all no-one else would be able to. The suggestion that breaking a difficulty into parts might mean that it is indeed soluble carries the implied criticism that relatives have attempted less than they might. This is a common reason for the 'I've tried that' phenomenon. However, this often means that relatives have only tried the solution on one occasion, and perhaps in adverse circumstances.

Once relatives have been able to carry out manoeuvres that have led to a beneficial change, however small, they have commenced the process of moving from negative to positive action; this signals the beginning of a shift from denial, avoidance and being weighed down by their circumstances. Relatives are now able to trust that the therapist's more optimistic view is right, and that, if things go wrong, it is possible with help to pick up the pieces.

This whole process can be quite time-consuming. It requires that the therapist projects an unthreatening image, does not appear too enthusiastic, and is prepared to tolerate the brickbats thrown by relatives from time to time. It is crucially important for therapists not to allow themselves to be shut out.

Grief

As discussed earlier, grieving is an apposite term to apply to people still in the early stages of coming to terms with the fact of mental illness in a relative. Parents must often mourn the loss of potential seen in a loved son or daughter. The hopes and aspirations that parents have for their children will reach their fruition in the adult; often these illnesses become apparent just as offspring are beginning to make an independent life. In consequence education may be disrupted, exams failed, jobs discontinued, relationships broken off. Thus much of the achievement hoped for from the child is likely to be blighted. A particularly bitter aspect of these long-term illnesses is that, even after recovery from the acute stage, negative symptoms like poor motivation, loss of interest, and poor concentration persist and conspire to prevent the son or daughter reestablishing anything like their old, pre-illness pattern of behaviour. One mother described it as 'his shattered life'.

With today's smaller families, it may be an only child, or an only son or daughter who becomes ill. Thus, much of the hope focused on the child is confounded. Even when there is more than one child in the family, comparison with their more successful siblings can be upsetting for both relatives and patients.

The grief is similar to that found in bereavement, with the exception that instead of a memory of a young healthy child, parents are faced with the reality of a middle aged son or daughter with a variety of problems, continuing to need a large amount of care and supervision and comparing unfavourably with other adults in the home. Creer et al. (1982) found that 30% of relatives provided physical care (washing, help with laundry, self-care) and other practical assistance (such as with budgeting) that most adults do not require.

Thus the bereavement is compounded: not only a process of loss, but also the requirement to adjust to a 'new' and often less appealing person. This is clearly evinced in the quotation on p. 79.

Partners must face a different sort of loss. Usually when they met and went on to make a commitment, the later problems were not particularly in evidence. When illness subsequently creates difficulties, which in the long-term group do not resolve easily, the partner faces not only the loss of a confidante, but also the fact that many of the other person's roles will be lost or grossly altered. For instance if patients were formerly employed, it may be months or years before they are ready to work again, if ever: the role status and financial advantage will all be foregone. Patients with other roles, such as housekeeping or childcare, may no longer be capable of carrying them out, wholly or in part. This usually means that, as well as 'losing' their partners, spouses have to take over these roles: they may have to get a job after a gap of many years or take on housework, childcare, or financial management. Joint decision-making often becomes a thing of the past — patients may lose all interest in domestic issues, or else make unilateral, often unrealistic decisions.

Grief thus becomes focused not only on the lost potential of the partner, but also on a relationship that can no longer develop as initially hoped. We have known no relative in this situation who has not considered separation or divorce. Often the relationship will break down — the divorce rate of married people who develop serious psychotic illnesses is considerably elevated.

Ordinary bereavement can be longlasting, and the sense of loss and sadness is mixed in with other emotions like rage, anger, helplessness, depression. The grief of the relatives of those with severe mental illness is frequently very prolonged indeed, since the provocation is continuous rather than a single event. It is also frequently compounded with other emotions, particularly if the current condition of patients shows great disparity with their former state. In order to assist relatives who are grieving in this way, the therapist must help them to see something positive in patients as they are now. If discussions cannot be moved away from how good things used to be before the illness, the relatives' frustration and hopelessness will be increased. Moreover this will renew the patients' sense of failure and emphasize the unattainability of their earlier aims; they are often too well aware that their previous life style and aspirations are no longer within reach. Some patients however go along with their relatives' nostalgia, and still try to fulfill expectations that may have been feasible before the illness developed; thus they may continue to look for jobs or girlfriends, to sit for exams, or to try living in a flat, in a way that lacks any realistic appraisal of how difficult such goals have become.

If patients and relatives are both aiming unrealistically high, staff will find it very difficult to engage the family. Even if they manage this first step, it will be almost impossible to negotiate practicable goals. The suggestion by staff that some small and feasible innovation should be attempted is rejected by the family, who, in strenuously denying reality, will see it as a slight. In this situation both patients and relatives need considerable help in understanding the illness and its effects, and education spread over many months may be required.

More commonly, patients will be aware that ordinary goals have become more difficult to achieve, as they have first hand experience of the disabling effects of their symptoms. However, they may find it very hard to communicate this clearly to relatives. They are then left open to blame, and may be labelled as 'lazy' or 'feckless' as relatives try feverishly to set up jobs or other adult activities, only to see patients fail or decline the opportunity.

Such relatives are effectively denying their loss — they refuse to countenance the inability of patients to fulfill their aspirations and hopes. The result is behaviour that appears grossly unrealistic to an outsider. Denying the patients' loss of function means denying that there is much of a problem, certainly not one that couldn't be sorted out with a bit more 'effort' from the patient.

Sometimes relatives shift the blame on to staff, who are seen as incompetent, unhelpful and obstructive because they have not cured the patient and made the problems disappear. Particularly with the general emphasis on the effectiveness of health care, there is an implicit assumption that professionals will be able to provide successful treatment. Relatives of long-term patients may consequently feel that if staff had acted earlier or done things differently, current difficulties would not have occurred.

Thus in the early stages, intervention may need to be devoted to helping patients and relatives face up to loss. Patients and relatives require the time and trust to discuss exactly what has happened, how devastating it feels and how upsetting it has been. While it is necessary to talk with families realistically, it is also possible to give them the support of knowing that their loss is not *total*: patients are still alive and have qualities that are important. They may still be able to offer relationships of some kind, and their life may still be a contribution rather than a mere drain on the relatives' resources.

If this perspective can be gained, not only can relatives feel a new, albeit partial, optimism, but patients may possibly regain a role in the family beyond being and feeling a burden. When they have recovered from the more acute stages of the illness, many patients are only too aware of the difficulties carers face, and this can add to their own low self esteem and feelings of depression.

Guilt

It is almost inevitable that carers faced with the realities of a long-term illness should search for a cause. They seek certainties, but professionals can only offer them generalities and are unable to be clear about the exact influences that have brought about the illness in individual patients. Carers therefore tend to retain their own version of what brought on the patients' problems (Berkowitz et al., 1984). Thus they often continue to feel that the problems must somehow have arisen, at least partially, because of their own failings.

The consequence of this is commonly a continual going back over the patient's early life in an attempt to discern the cause. Relatives may actualy be able to pinpoint some event that they feel must have contributed, for instance, parental divorce. In other cases, the putative cause is more nebulous — perhaps not spending enough time with or not being close enough to the patient in childhood.

The guilt concerned with distant causes is a particularly demoralizing emotion. Even if identifiable past events were significant, there is nothing that can be done about them. The consequence is an unproductive harping on the past, which often includes a continual and often unrealistic rehearsal of how things were before they went wrong. This involves denial of the earlier imperfections of relationships and situations in a manner that operates against any commitment to changing things in the present.

Such feelings are closely connected with overinvolvement, and as such are more characteristic of parents than spouses. However, spouses may feel guilty too, often reproaching themselves for not being sympathetic enough.

These comments apply to guilt about the past. Guilt about present circumstances is also common, and one of its most frequent objects is social activity. Many long-term patients withdraw socially, and relatives then feel guilty about not including them in their own socializing — this despite the fact that patients are obviously avoiding opportunities of this type. In consequence, relatives may dragoon patients into accompanying them. The clear realization that patients have not enjoyed the outing makes them feel more guilty still. Alternatively, relatives will leave patients at home, and feel guilty about having done so, particularly if they actually manage to enjoy themselves a little.

These common difficulties over their social lives form part of the reason why relatives often become very socially isolated indeed. They arise from ignorance of the nature of the patients' social withdrawal, that it is in fact a symptom of their illness, and may within limits have a positive function for them.

There are several principles that should govern the attempts of staff to deal with guilt — it certainly needs dealing with as it is so destructive, gnawing away at carers without permitting them to do anything constructive.

First, professionals must be seen to be receptive. They must believe that guilt is very upsetting to relatives, and that it is worthwhile to spend time listening to them. Secondly, they must provide a perspective by letting relatives know that the feelings that are causing them anguish are actually very common and that others have experienced them before. Thirdly, professionals need to be firm about moving relatives on, getting them to do things that are constructive, however they feel, and using the concern that guilt reflects in a more productive way. Fourthly, it is probably fair to say, and certainly good to say to relatives, that, of all the causes contributing to the emergence of schizophrenia and other severe mental illnesses, the style of parenting will be of little importance. After all, many people experience parental divorce without becoming mad.

The final principle requires the reframing or redirection of overinvolvement. So, for example, it can be suggested that in the context of these illnesses, it may be as caring to allow patients to have time of their own as it is to provide them with social outlets they may not relish, or to remain cooped up with them all the livelong day. It is important to 'give permission' for carers to have a life of their own.

Fear of the Future

Many carers have fears about the future, in particular if they are the elderly parents of patients: 'what will happen when I'm gone?'. The fear often represents a realistic appraisal of the vulnerabilities of the patient and of the irreplaceable quality of care provided by relatives. Sometimes however it is not possible for staff to evaluate how realistic the fears are, as the patients' assets may be obscured by a dependency fostered by their domestic situation.

Ideally, the potentialities of patients should be tested by enlisting the relatives' help in encouraging an increasing independence. It can be emphasized that it is appropriate to get patients to do more for themselves while relatives are still capable of providing back up if necessary. If things go well relatives may then obtain the reassurance that comes from improvement. It is also reassuring if relatives are made aware that the teams' involvement will continue.

Using change in this way may nevertheless be difficult in the long-term mentally ill. They and their relatives may be locked in very rigid patterns, and either parent or patient may refuse to cooperate. Some families may just be content to stay largely as they are, and realistic appraisal then has to wait until a parent dies. On the other hand, if parents become ill or frail, it may then be possible gradually to increase the patients' scope for independence. Staff must be alert to these opportunities, as reassurance has particular value to carers who have become less able to care and know that they probably do not have that long to live.

Anger and Rejection of the Patient

Both relatives and staff members may be angered by patients. This is usually because of specific aspects of their behaviour, such as shouting abuse, hitting out, or refusal to cooperate with treatment. Carers can be at the end of their tether because patients persist in doing things they find intolerable. This behaviour often lacks an obvious connection with their illness. For instance, it may take the form of common abuse or getting frequently drunk. Staff may also feel demoralized and helpless in the face of longstanding violent or objectionable behaviour.

One of the problems that arises from the anger of carers and staff members is that it gets displaced: carers become angry with staff, staff with carers. Relatives blame the staff for not doing more, or for not intervening earlier or more effectively. Staff feel angry with relatives because they suspect they are making things worse. Patients are seldom passive observers — if these splits occur, they may play both ends against the middle, sometimes very effectively indeed.

In extreme cases, patients may be thrown out of the house (or hostel!), and staff then feel that they have been landed with a difficult problem that might have been avoided.

How then to deal with this anger? One of its origins is a feeling of personal responsibility for patients' behaviour and a sense of frustration at being unable to handle it better. It therefore helps considerably if the protagonists can stand back and avoid seeing the patients' problems as their own personal failure. Aims with long-term patients may need to be modest, and it may be that little progress is possible. However, this cannot really be seen as anyone's fault.

Staff should also try to distinguish what is under the patients' control, even if incompletely so. It may then be possible to get them to give up their most infuriating actions. Otherwise, it may be necessary to consider a change in the level of medication or a structured alteration in the environment. Above all, staff, provided they are aware of what is going on, should take the initiative in calling a halt to the process of mutual recrimination with relatives. Relatives also need to be persuaded that they have no grounds for feeling personally responsible for patients' bad behaviour. It is helpful if staff and carers can accept that it is all right to be angry, but acknowledge the necessity for separating the anger from the way they deal with patients. Above all, it should not affect their treatment — a counsel of perfection, but an essential aspiration.

In some cases, carers remain so angry and frustrated with patients that they eventually reject them, perhaps refusing to remain in contact. Staff obviously have to accept such decisions, which may merely be a true recognition of the reality of the situation. In some cases, the distancing effected by the patient moving from the parental home may actually allow carers to provide care at a lesser level, but less distorted by powerful emotions on both sides.

Sometimes anger is the result of a specific incident, rather than the result of continuing turmoil at home or in relation to services. In this case a debriefing session is needed, with relatives or with other staff members according to the nature and location of the incident. The exact circumstances should be established, followed by a discussion of ways in which the incident might have been handled differently and the development of contingency plans to avoid repetition. Likewise, there should be a constructive attempt to delineate limits.

Where individual staff members are working with very difficult patients, support from colleagues is absolutely essential. They should not work in isolation, and they should not be left to deal with overwhelming problems alone. They must have the sense that responsibility is shared. A multidisciplinary team is the most obvious method of sharing the responsibility and support and, at the very least, staff should have access to this back-up (Bennett, 1983).

8·Problem Solving

Problem solving is a universal human activity that can be enhanced by making particular strategies more explicit. Finding and implementing wise solutions to problems is the hallmark of a good therapist, but transmitting this ability to clients is an even more important function. This applies particularly when the clients are caring for those with enduring and severe psychiatric illnesses. Their lives are a sea of problems, and are made so partly because their attempts at solving them are not very successful.

A major function of those working with the families faced with severe mental illness is thus to increase the families' ability to find a solution to their difficulties and, one way or another, to ensure that the burden of problems is reduced. The objective is to improve the functioning of the family as a unit.

Many families have problems, and some are so common as to be almost a characteristic of family living — marital discord, intergenerational communication difficulties, sibling rivalry. However, these problems may be more apparent and more difficult to deal with when they are complicated by mental illness in a family member. This may increase the difficulties relatives have in expressing their feelings, or make it harder for them to defuse tension. Indeed, mental illness effectively changes the rules of the game so that ordinary strategies of coping are no longer applicable or successful. Ignorance about the nature of the condition multiplies the difficulties. In effect, mental illness in the family makes problem solving itself a problem.

Moreover, as we have emphasized throughout this book, mental illness brings new problems for families. These include stigma, social isolation, the need to readjust role allocation, and difficult behaviour on the patients' part that does not seem to respond to commonsense methods of dealing with it.

General Principles

In this chapter, we shall discuss some of the difficulties experienced by therapists in dealing with the problems of families with mentally ill members, and in getting family members to adopt more effective methods of addressing their problems themselves. Effective interventions are often hard to identify and to implement, and it may sometimes be impossible to find a solution at all. Nevertheless, a pragmatic and structured approach greatly increases the chance of success.

Before dealing with difficult issues specific to this client group, we will therefore outline the principles involved in solving problems and enhancing such skills in others.

Problem solving may be ineffective for a number of reasons. First, members of the family may not be very good at communicating with each other and with the therapist. Secondly, they may choose inappropriate solutions, and finally they may not implement the chosen solution in a manner likely to bring success.

There are a number of ways in which people may show an impaired ability to communicate. The deficits may be relatively gross, arising from deficient non-verbal elements like poor eye contact, or a facial expression that is inappropriate in some way. However, the deficits may be revealed at a higher level of functioning. There is evidence that high Expressed Emotion in the relatives of patients with schizophrenia is associated with deficiency in higher level skills (Kuipers et al., 1983). Such relatives tend to be poor listeners, interrupting and often talking across patients, and sometimes the therapist. In addition, they may not allow patients to speak for themselves, and describe their feelings or opinions without confirming them. Some make a habit of publicly invalidating the patients' experiences and feelings. They may give mixed messages, and sometimes make demands in a threatening and coercive manner. Finally, they often talk at a tangent to the subject in hand, a clear disadvantage in the attempt to address problematic issues.

If there is evidence of inappropriate communication of this type, the therapist must attempt to deal with it. Even small gains may permit families and therapists to engage more constructively in seeking the solution of problems. First, the nature of the impairments in communication skills must be identified. Are clients poor listeners, cutting across other people and not giving them space to make their feelings known? Or do they communicate in a vague way, being given to self contradiction or overgeneralization? Do they communicate in a destructive way, making hostile or overcritical remarks. Are they poor at conveying positive feelings?

Listening skills involve non-verbal indications of attentiveness (uh-huh, eye contact, and so on), and responsive questioning aimed at clarification. Clarification may be required both about facts and feelings, and it is also useful to paraphrase or otherwise check that messages have been received correctly. The most effective way of increasing the listening skills of family members is by intervening when they interrupt, by making direct invitations to them to listen to the other person, and by modelling good listening practices.

A vague communication style is best modified by clarificatory questioning and by pointing out inconsistencies in such a way that the real message can be winkled out. It also requires the therapist to reinforce clients for being able to get a specific message across, by responding to it seriously. This is essentially a shaping procedure, and it takes time to modify the client's actual style. However, in the process, enough specific communication is effected for the therapist to be able to work on.

Destructive communication obliges the therapist to take control of the interaction. Criticism is most destructive when expressed with heat, or in general terms as criticism of the person as a whole. The therapist can take away some of the heat and the overgenerality by relaxed exploration leading to a formulation of specific requests for change. Again, the therapist can point out the usefulness and constructiveness of the end result. This may encourage a better style of communication in the relative, and this may even generalize to the home situation, when the therapist is not there. However, criticism has complicated origins, and it may require other changes in the family before it abates significantly.

Finally, families may not be very rewarding to each other — they may not be very good at saying when they are pleased with each other. The best way to change this is for the therapist to point out to relatives when something good has been achieved and to model the communication of pleasure. This requires the therapist to identify some occurrence or action as good. The good aspects may not at first be apparent to relatives, so this identification process may help them to adjust their attributions of the event in a helpful way. The next part of the process is for therapists to make their own pleasure clear to the family, perhaps in a way designed to invite them to agree. The process of problem solving will itself result in material that can be used in sesssions in this way.

The first prerequisite for solving a problem is to *define* it. In some cases, the families' difficulties may largely reflect a degree of incompetence in pinpointing what the problem is. This is obviously a considerable bar to dealing with it. It requires clarification through gentle cross-examination by the therapist, who will thus be modelling an effective approach to problem definition. The important aspects need to be identified and irrelevancies discarded. In some cases or in later stages, the therapist may be able to get the family to carry out the process of clarification themselves. This may be easier where the family has more members.

For the therapist, the next step involves an evaluation of the problem, a 'functional analysis' in the language of behaviour therapy. This means getting some idea of the place of the problem in the economy of the family: how is the family handicapped by the problem, what does each member gain from the existence of the problem, what would they gain from its removal or reduction, what things seem to influence the frequency of the problem, what are the typical triggers? This should be done in some detail. Once done the therapist will know something of the approach to adopt and the chances of success.

The next part of the process of problem-solving is the identification of a series of potential solutions. Very often, families may not be very imaginative in doing this, and the strengths of a good therapist include being able to provide a dimension of lateral thinking to their deliberations.

The next step is a consideration of the advantages and disadvantages of alternative solutions, without immediately plumping for an obvious front runner. All solutions should be taken seriously, even if they are regarded by some of those present as a bit daft. After all, the best solution may not turn out to be the most obvious. It is worthwhile to reinforce all attempts at a constructive contribution even when the suggestion appears unrealistic from the first.

After this, a decision about the best solution or combinations of solutions must be taken, and plans must be made about how it shall be implemented. These should be specified in some detail, with the responsibilities of each member of the family spelt out.

The required action may need to be spread over several stages. Poor implementation is often the reason for continuing difficulties. A date should be set by which initiatives should have been attempted, although usually this can be done informally by telling the family that the therapist will ask them about progress at the next appointment:

The final element in effective problem-solving is a review of progress. Sometimes progress will have been good or at any rate fair, and this is the opportunity for the therapist to reinforce the constructiveness of relatives' attempts to change things. Failure will often have to be addressed. The therapist needs to know the reasons for it. These include inadequate effort, which may result if the task was too difficult or some members of the family did not understand or agree with what was decided. Other things may genuinely have diverted the energies of the family, but sometimes the attempt has been sabotaged by one or more family members. The reasons for this also need to be teased out in a delicate way.

Failure sometimes results despite the families' best efforts. This may be because the wrong problem or the wrong solution was chosen, and both these possibilities should be reviewed. Sometimes, the problem has not been broken down enough for action. The therapist should always attempt to see something positive in the families' attempts, and to provide them with this reinterpretation.

In parallel with these attempts at solving difficulties, the therapist requires to rehearse the possible consequences, particularly the bad ones. Some of the resistance of families towards addressing their difficulties arises from a fear of making things worse, and this may be realistic. The fear can be controlled by providing a safety net which would include various ways, emotional, intellectual and practical, of dealing with possible disappointments. Forewarned is forearmed.

These approaches to problem solving are essentially behavioural and represent a development of ideas on behavioural problem solving by Spivak and his colleagues (1976). They are spelled out in more detail by Falloon and his colleagues (1984), who used them in a highly structured family therapy intervention with a sample of schizophrenic patients.

In our view, the benefit of this approach lies in the structure it provides. However, we feel that for the long-term group of patients an over-rigid adherence to this structure in the practice of therapy may be counterproductive. This does not mean that the structure should not shape the way we think about patients, relatives and their problems, just that the principles may need to be implemented with subtlety and delicacy.

Solving Problems with the Relatives of Those with Longstanding Mental Illness

This group may present the therapist with a wide variety of problems, ranging from the mundane and specific — getting someone to eat every day, to look after their hygiene adequately, to manage a budget a little better — to more complex issues, such as why someone cannot lead a more independent life, why they sabotage attempts to get them better, and so on.

It is particularly necessary in this group to separate the soluble from the insoluble. The therapist should resist the obligation to solve everything. After all, families will have been dealing with their situation for many years and have come at least to some kind of adjustment — the consequence is that many aspects are unlikely to change greatly or easily.

There are clear dangers in choosing the wrong problem as a target, for instance, a problem that no-one wants solved, or that is being reinforced in a way that makes change unlikely. Getting a young man to attend a day centre may be resisted strenuously if it means his mother must face an even greater degree of isolation. If therapists do make a wrong choice, it allows families to disregard them, to denigrate their status and contribution, and perhaps, to cast them aside as a waste of time and effort, while retaining a sense of self-righteousness.

It therefore behoves the therapist to select an initial target that is relatively specific and isolated, and appears amenable to change. Even if this is done carefully, there is of course still no guarantee that it will indeed be soluble. Family members sometimes offer up as soluble something that looks reasonably simple, but actually turns out to have been, all along, a major sticking point that no-one can do anything about. The wily therapist may be able to spot this and opt for a different target. The chance of doing this is increased if a whole range of problems is examined before one is decided upon. If it rapidly transpires that a wrong decision has been made, the therapist must be flexible enough to move on to another problem, and avoid the counterproductive banging of heads against brick walls.

That insoluble problems exist seems not to be a popular view: however, it is essential to recognize that this is so when working with the relatives of the long-term mentally ill. The therapist who feels obliged to solve every problem will very soon feel the capacity of families for being obstructive.

Significant change will only come about if families allow therapists some purchase on the problem. If they will not let them get to grips with it, therapists may just have to accept that that is the way things are. Timing is of crucial importance here: something that appears insoluble now may be more capable of alteration in a year or so, particularly if circumstances have changed a little in other ways. The therapist then has to be alert to the possibility of returning to ground that has seemed infertile in the past. So, for example, a family may operate on the fixed basis that the mother does everything, her ill son nothing. The mother's increasing frailty may permit the therapist to encourage the son to do more, develop greater skills and autonomy and have his efforts genuinely valued. If the opportunity is not spotted, however, it will go to waste. This underlines the need for continual review.

Some situations are only problems at all because of the way they are defined. The role of the therapist in facilitating a redefinition of the situation may actually render it unproblematic. It is thus relevant to ask who defines what a problem is, for whom is it a problem, and why has it become defined as a problem.

Sometimes relatives will propose as a problem what is really its cause. So, for instance, a mother may complain that her son does not take baths, when the real issue is the fact that he is dirty and unkempt. If this is realized, it is possible to see that the solution is not primarily to get him to take baths, but to increase his general level of cleanliness. This then opens the door to other possible interventions, like getting him to strip-wash rather than bathe, or arranging for him to be supervised in bathing at a day facility. In general, dealing with effects rather than causes increases the range of options.

We have mentioned the importance of deficiencies in listening skills, and these may be particularly apparent and relevant among the relatives of the long-term group of patients. They may be very disparate, ranging from talking too much to talking too little. Relatives may be very poor indeed at allowing patients space to express themselves, or at being able to tolerate another viewpoint. They may have become used to speaking for or speaking over patients, or even shouting them down. The skill of the therapist there involves getting families to allow patients a valid representation.

In some cases, however, it is the patient who does not listen; relatives may have been cowed over many years by patients given to forceful self-expression, and in consequence may have had to put up with a continual reiteration of mad opinions and beliefs.

Situations where one member of the family is dominating the interaction require firm action by the therapist. Interruptions cannot be tolerated, and must be gently but firmly discouraged. The therapist should take charge of the conversation so that family members can speak turn and turn about. Neither can relatives be allowed to speak for patients or other family members. The therapist must control this, either by introjecting directly, or by feeding back the inappropriateness of this behaviour. The way the therapist deals with the patient is crucial here, as it provides a powerful model for an alternative style of interaction — listening attentively, ignoring or setting limits on mad talk, pulling out the sensible elements from perhaps largely unrealistic contributions.

If patients insist on talking about hallucinations or delusions, the therapist should attempt to get them to acknowledge how distressing they are. This again permits the separation of sane responses from mad experiences and beliefs, and allows the therapist to respond to them differentially, reinforcing one and not the other.

In our practice, some families are immigrants with a different culture of communication. In Cypriot families, for instance, it may be the tradition for the senior male to do the talking for the family. This may in any case lead to conflict between the generations, as the British born younger members may attempt to move to a different and more egalitarian pattern. Whilst acknowledging the validity of other cultural traditions, we have found it easier to work with families when this particular pattern of a single dominant member has been attenuated. We have therefore tended to try to bring this about through the manner of our intervention; clearly, this must be done with care and an appreciation of the sensibilities of each family member. One must avoid seeming to threaten the status of the dominant member too crudely. In working with these families one may nevertheless have to accept a circumscribed success.

In the process of assessing difficulties, it is important not to accept the families' agenda uncritically. The overall situation of families must be evaluated before a decision is taken about what should be targetted. If families quite clearly feel that one particular problem is the main one and must be dealt with, the therapist must strike a balance between accepting that for the family it is a source and focus of real distress and therefore important, and declining to deal with something that will not be readily shifted at an early stage. The therapist should be prepared to listen, acknowledge the associated distress, and find out why the family thinks it wants the problem dealt with. This should lead on to a further dissection of the problem. Breaking the problem down in this way is a prerequisite to identifying manageable targets, but also carries the advantage of allowing the therapist to decline to focus on solving the problem presented while appearing to take the issue seriously. The process of listening and of letting the families say how bad it all is sometimes results in them 'taking the problem back' and saying that they can cope with it. It is as if the main need was for the problem to be paraded.

The consequence of not giving time to hear about the panoply of problems is to appear as though disparaging or denigrating their reality. If families feel the therapist is doing this, the problem will brought back time and again. It will also grow, being presented as larger on each occasion.

Among the relatives of the long-term group, the process of listening may need to be prolonged. It may indeed be some time before relatives will let the therapist in so he or she can actually facilitate changes in their situation.

Once therapists have heard through all the problems, they have, so to speak, earned the right to move on with the family to the actuality of making things change. They are now entitled to focus on the specifics of a single problem.

Even this act of focusing carries implications. It suggests first that change is possible, and secondly that things might actually be made worse. The implied possibility of change is often seen as a criticism of families' previous efforts, and people coping at the margins of their resourcefulness may not be able to contemplate the possibility of a worsening situation. In either case the response is likely to be obstructive. Focusing must therefore be done very carefully and supportively. Considerable time may be needed here, and the therapist may have to spend fifteen minutes on, say, the exact procedures involved in buying a tin of cat food. It is useful to say something like 'if there had been an easy solution, you would have found it'. All sorts of reasons may be given for arguing that some situations are beyond rectification. An important part of the therapist's function is to field these objections. Sometimes relatives will say 'it won't make any difference'. Under these circumstances it helps to emphasize that rapid change is not looked for, but this is no reason for not trying. Likewise targets should represent small manageable steps — setting easy targets makes a degree of success more likely. It is very important to get families to realize they can change their approach to things. Moderating the expectations of highly critical relatives may be a prerequisite to this. Sometimes the therapist may have to agree that a problem is not in fact soluble.

Once a problem has been selected for attention, the various stages described above can be traversed. It is important to negotiate a solution that incorporates patients' views, and even better if they can be persuaded to contribute some possible solutions. This may be difficult for some members of the long-term group.

Sometimes the solution will involve *encouraging* behaviour — enhancing motivation and the like; on other occasions it is concerned with *preventing* certain behaviours, setting limits and so on.

Setting home work tasks is crucial, as most changes concern circumstances at home that are impossible to deal with outside. The exact nature of the task objective must be specified. The setting of tasks ensures a focus for discussion at the next visit. Whatever comes back is of use.

The consequences of attempts at change can be myriad and the therapist can end up being quite surprised at the information that is fed back. An apparent obstructiveness at an earlier session may not stop families from approaching and even solving the target problem. In a way, this provides a victory 'for both sides' — the therapist's intervention has been successful but the family have not relinquished their autonomy to the professionals. Indeed, if they so wish, they can still feel that their success was nothing at all to do with the therapist. The therapist, if wise, will go along with this. The role of the therapist is sometimes just to give families the confidence to try their own thing; this may be an approach quite different from that arrived at in negotiations towards tentative solutions. The therapist should nevertheless reinforce the success, however arrived at.

On other occasions, families may present the problem at a subsequent meeting as really being quite trivial, not at all as important as it was first made out to be. In some cases, this is an attempt to discount their own successes. The technique here is to go back over the situation and their actions in detail, and get relatives to see and acknowledge the progress they have made. (Don't let them get away with it!)

In other cases, it is possible that what was presented as a big problem was actually relatively trivial, but was presented knowingly as a sort of 'try-on' by the relatives. In such circumstances, therapists should not spend too much time over the issue: they should acknowledge the success gracefully, but then move on to something more significant.

As families manage to deal with even quite small problems, leading to quite small changes, life may become a little easier. Patients may be doing more or behaving better, but a major component of the relaxation is the change in attitudes fostered by the very attempt at altering things. Obviously attempts at facilitating problem solving do not take place in a therapeutic vacuum. There are other things going on in family meetings and group meetings — ventilation, emotional processing, support — and if these various aspects can be harnessed together the effects can be quite marked. Managing to achieve this synergy demands considerable skill from the therapist, but is most rewarding.

The therapist must be prepared to take things slowly without being discouraged. There often needs to be a lot of repetitiveness in work with these families. Sometimes aims may have to be lowered: intervention may be about damage limitation, or at best making things manageable. So, for instance, it may not be possible to stop patients hitting out, but it may be possible to limit the effects and keep people reasonably safe.

Not all problems can be dealt with within the resources of the family. It is possible for example, that certain practical difficulties can only be overcome through the special access of the therapist to other resources. The therapist may consequently be called on to act in the role of almoner, organizing debt counselling through the Citizen's Advice Bureau, dealing with housing departments or associations, setting up a home help, getting certain bills paid directly through the benefit system, or getting in the 'dirty squad'. Involvement in such activities is a two edged sword: it pleases the family that the therapist is prepared to put in the effort and it may provide a launchpad for other types of change, but it may not encourage the family to do as much as they can for themselves.

Insoluble Problems

As we have suggested on various occasions above, some problems are insoluble. It is extremely important for staff to recognize the limitations of the possible and not to take a lack of success personally. It means they will have to live under the burden of insoluble problems, but families of long-term mental patients have to do that anyway. Indeed, taking on some of the burden of such problems is part of the function of a service for those with longstanding illnesses. Ultimately, staff have to accept the right of patients not to deal with a particular difficulty — they may live in very squalid conditions, but yet be constructive in other ways.

Some insoluble problems operate as a sort of currency — they enable a patient to buy into a service. Staff often get very worried by patients whom they suspect of using problems in this way, although there comes a point where flagrant demands indicate genuine need. Dealing with such cases requires a policy of damage limitation, usually managed by insisting that all requests are dealt with through a single key worker. The rest of the multidisciplinary team have a bounden duty to be alert to the requirement of providing support for colleagues who have taken on this role — they will need it.

As we have suggested above, there are many aspects of working with the long-term group that contribute to staff 'burn out'. This is minimized by the proper working of a multidisciplinary team (see p. 18).

Within limits, it can also be good for therapists to allow patients and their families to see that they have been upset. It models openness and sharing, it is good for them to feel that they have a contribution to make and are not always on the receiving end, and they may be quite supportive. Indeed, relatives are often very good at this; they have frequently had plenty of practice. On the other hand, therapists would be unwise to expect families to mop them up in any major way.

9·Helping with Specific Issues

In previous chapters we have been concerned more with the principles and strategy of intervening with relatives in the management of the long-term group. Although in the process we have touched directly on how clinicians might deal with several practical problems, staff members are often fearful of working with relatives because they do not feel competent to answer the practical queries of relatives. In this chapter we provide guidelines that have proved useful for responding to common queries of this type.

Dealing with Apathy

Staff need to be clear that loss of energy, sleeping a lot, spending time doing nothing and wanting to avoid people are common after-effects of a severe mental illness. As discussed earlier however, these are most likely to be misattributed by relatives and seen primarily as laziness and unfriendliness on the patients' part. Even after many years of contact, staff may have to resign themselves to a difference of opinion, as some relatives can never really be brought to believe in negative symptoms. Nevertheless if some tolerance and acceptance of the lessened activity level can be communicated, much of the anger and frustration elicited by the patient's apathy can be defused. In family meetings, patients can often be helped to describe the feelings of pointlessness and deadness that often accompany the lack of activity and thus give some reason for it; although some patients may only be able to talk of being tired all the time.

While some of the problems are due to misattribution, patients who do nothing *at all* but sit in one room risk losing skills and confidence. Thus some minimal, functional level of activity should be negotiated with the whole family and gradually built upon through the problem solving techniques described in Chapter 8. Again the pace and expectation of change must be realistic, and staff may need to help the family to take a very long-term perspective — over a year, or even five. While it may be sensible to negotiate that patients spend some time on their own, too much isolation must be discouraged, perhaps by setting 'homework tasks' such as staying in the living room (even if not speaking) when visitors arrive, or accompanying relatives to a social occasion, even if participation is rather passive. Levels of activity must be gradually increased as competence and interest return, and patients who needed constant prompting even to do the washing up may eventually be persuaded to go out on their own or to manage the shopping.

It is common for a lack of energy and social withdrawal to lead patients to stay in bed of a morning. Staff and relatives may find this difficult to deal with. Again it is helpful to be clear, to negotiate expectations and then consistently apply the practice. For instance it can be sensible for staff and family to work out what is a reasonable time to aim at, and then how to offer prompts without confrontation. One family offered time checks and cups of tea, but not breakfast, which remained downstairs: this was after a time for getting up had been agreed between carers and patient (10.00 am). Once it has been possible to establish this sort of arrangement, an earlier time of rising can be negotiated, provided there is something for the patient to get up for.

Self-care

Severe mental illness, particularly where there are many negative symptoms, may significantly impair self-care. In extreme cases, self-neglect may be severe, patients do not eat properly and live in squalor. Even if they live with relatives, there are frequently day-to-day problems over bathing or shaving, and there may be a difficulty about changing clothes, particularly underwear. One mother described how her son became attached to the particular set of clothes he had on and would not change them. All she could do was to persuade him to bathe about once a month, and to wash these clothes while he was doing so. When eventually they wore out, the same thing happened to the new set.

In these circumstances it is helpful for staff to establish with the family a *minimum* frequency of, say bathing, laundering, and changing of sheets that is at any rate tolerable, both to carer and patient. Once a week may be a reasonable target, and, once negotiated, staff should encourage relatives and patients to continue with it. It can be useful if one day of the week can be targeted as convenient. It may also be a good idea to suggest that the bathing is part of a general routine of getting up, getting dressed and getting out of the house. One of our patients particularly liked to attend the Day Centre on a Wednesday, and this was targeted as the day for a bath and change of clothes, as well as the day for going out. To start off with, self-care may well need practical intervention on the relatives' part; shaving or hairwashing may be particularly burdensome for patients who are feeling very pre-occupied or unwell. However, this level of personal care should not be continued by relatives unless circumstances are extreme: as far as possible the aim should be to help patients do the tasks for themselves, even if continued verbal prompting is required. If a lot of physical help is needed, it may be better for staff to provide it, rather than relatives.

Dealing with Unacceptable or Embarrassing Behaviour

While families vary in their tolerance, we know that there are several sorts of behaviour they are likely to find unacceptable. They may find it intolerable when patients shout, swear or talk to themselves in a rather obvious manner, damage furniture or other objects, or threaten to harm themselves or others. They will want to control behaviour like this, but are frequently unsure about the best way to do so, without causing worse arguments or upsetting the patient. It is a counsel of perfection to advise relatives to remain calm. Nevertheless if they can do this, the benefits are considerable as becoming upset or angry just makes things worse.

It can be helpful if staff point out to carers that their relatives are not and were not always like this. Patients are often not aware of exactly how hurtful or upsetting their behaviour is, and may well be reacting in this way because they are actually very angry or frightened. After a particular outburst is over, it should be discussed once everyone has regained some tranquillity. It is often best to do this in a family session. It is important for relatives to acknowledge to patients that they may be frightened or upset and offer support, eg. 'I know you've been upset, what can I do to help?'. At the time it may be a good idea for relatives to leave the room, or to suggest that patients go to their own room for a while. One patient would often talk and swear to himself. After talking with staff the family managed to limit this by negotiating with the patient that when he needed to do this, he would go to his bedroom.

After a particularly upsetting or embarrassing event staff should invite patient and carers to a meeting so that everyone can discuss how it felt. If staff are there as mediators it is likely that anger and hurt can be expressed, and at the same time contained. It is helpful if all members of the family can be honest about what they felt, even if it is negative. The staff role in this is to enable negative emotions to be expressed without the more negative consequence of patients or carers withdrawing or becoming very angry. If anger and hurt can be expressed in a factual manner the effects of embarrassing behaviour can be discussed. It is then possible to begin to work out ways of limiting or avoiding similar situations in future. Without this sort of discussion patients and carers may have no mutual insight in to the effect of their behaviour on each other. As part of the discussion staff should help the family make clear both what causes the behaviour and what can be tolerated, so that in future incidents may be defused.

One man when severely ill would take his clothes off, regardless of who else was in the room. His mother and married sister, who lived with him, were encouraged to ask him when he was less psychotic why he did this. They also told him how upsetting it was for them. He said that sometimes his voices told him to undress as an act of penitence, and that he was unaware of its effect on them, although when severely ill he was in any case unable to control this behaviour. He was eventually able to agree to do it in private whenever possible, although he needed reminding. Nevertheless the strategy worked reasonably well, both because his relatives understood and thus could sympathize with his need to act in his way, and because, having agreed to it previously, the patient could respond to prompting even when very disturbed.

Coping with Delusions

Many relatives find it difficult to know how to respond to delusions, particularly if they are strongly expressed. If they deny the truth of the delusion, they may be seen to have 'joined the enemy'. If they go along with it, the belief becomes even more fixed in the sufferer's mind. Arguing is not helpful.

With this problem, staff need to help relatives to draw the line. It is appropriate for relatives to sympathize with the distress the delusion may cause and to agree that the belief is real for the patient, but they must then make it clear that the experience is *not* real for them. This not only offers support to the patient, but also helps them to understand where they differ from others over what is reality. For example if a patient is convinced that the TV is sending direct messages, the relative can say 'I know you think the TV is talking to you, you are sensitive to that sort of thing at times, I don't find it talks to me' and this distinguishes between the patient's own reality and that of other people.

Patients will often experience considerable relief when it is made clear for instance that their thoughts are not in fact read by other people, even if the belief is fixed. In another example, a patient's wife could not at first understand what her husband was talking about when he said he was convinced that he had a special mission to fulfill. While agreeing with him and sympathizing that he felt such urgency, she made it clear that she did not share his belief, and that it was more important to her to have some help with a specific task (looking after their young son in this case). This combination of sympathy (it is very important for carers not to be dismissive) and distraction was often successful in calming him and helping him not to act on his belief.

Staff should suggest that relatives discourage patients from talking about delusions to anyone and everyone. It can be proposed to the patient that, in general, they do not have to talk about such things to people who are not staff or members of the immediate family. In fact, it is often a help to the family if a member of staff, usually the key worker, is delegated to listen to delusional beliefs. He or she may find it possible to offer specific support to the patient if delusions are very distressing, and to suggest strategies of dealing with them. They may also be able to encourage insight into the falsity of the beliefs, particularly during recovery from an acute episode or at times when insight in general may have improved.

Dealing with Unpredictability

Both staff and relatives may find unpredictable behaviour difficult to cope with. A patient may be 'her old self' for some days and then quite suddenly 'we lost her again'. There may be no warning of these mood changes so that an ordinary conversation can turn into a sudden series of accusations without apparent reason. Clinicians should emphasize to carers that such things occur in severe mental illnesses, and that patients are often not in control of these strong feelings that suddenly become convictions.

It can be helpful to alert carers both to the possibility of such changes and to their likely triggers, although these are not necessarily under the control of either relative or patient. Distraction is often the best strategy for this, eg. the carer or staff changes the subject and tries a more neutral topic. If unpredictability is a severe problem, it is likely to be brought up during a family meeting, and the staff member can then model a more appropriate strategy directly. This can be a powerful way of helping to change previously destructive interactions. One patient, who often started a 'tirade' against the Russians, could be deflected by the offer of a cup of tea. On other occasions, he would respond to the firm suggestion 'sit down until you feel calmer'.

If distraction is not possible, it may be better to encourage relative and patient to leave each other alone, until both can talk of something more neutral. This strategy overlaps with limit setting, and with coping with delusions, as reassurance may also be necessary if the patient is agitated or upset.

Restlessness, Overactivity and Anxiety

Some patients become extremely restless, uncomfortable and upset. They may be unable to sit still or to sleep, and spend hours pacing the room. No amount of reassurance seems to make any difference. Carers may find this behaviour almost unbearable if it continues for long, and so indeed may staff. Again, it is nearly always helpful to encourage relatives to make clear to patients that they realize how distressed they are. It is also appropriate for carers to communicate to patients how frustrating they themselves find their behaviour, although in a calm way: 'It upsets me to see you pacing the room like that'. It may be helpful to suggest a shared physical activity, perhaps a walk outside as a distraction. Otherwise it may be better for carers to leave the patient alone and relax on their own a little.

One of our patients would sometimes feel unbearably anxious and upset, and ask constantly for reassurance that 'it was not her fault' and that she was not shouting obscenities. This was very difficult for her family to tolerate, as indeed it was for the staff when she went into hospital: reassurance did no more than help her temporarily, and the feelings might last for days at a time. The best solution we could negotiate was to offer a brief stock phrase of reassurance plus some distraction. We avoided spending time trying to comfort her, and suggested the family did the same as it did not ease her distress but merely led to a great sense of frustration in those around her. Comments like 'we know how upset you are, try to sit down and watch TV/read the paper' seemed helpful while this distressing behaviour was at its height.

Coping with Violent Behaviour

Although relatively few mentally ill people are in any way violent, a minority of long-term patients may show a persistent tendency in this direction. This poses some rather special problems for the people who live with them.

The first thing for staff to acknowledge about violence is that, like suicide, it is not always preventable. There will sometimes be situations where it erupts without anyone being able to do anything to stop it. In the worst possible case, a pattern of repeated violence may be so established, for instance between a powerful son and his ageing frail mother, that it is not possible to change it. In such cases, it may be necessary for the sufferer and relative to stop living together, and even for the relative to take such actions as changing the locks or getting a court injunction against the offending person.

However, things are not usually that bad, and staff members may be able to suggest, and help to implement, action to deal with the violent behaviour. This action has three aspects, depending on whether it is to do with anticipating the violence, deals with the act itself, or takes place in the aftermath.

Effective action before someone actually behaves aggressively is obviously to be preferred. If staff and carers are aware that the patient is particularly irritable and therefore in a mood that may lead to violence, they may be able to avoid triggering it. It may be possible to increase this awareness by exploring with carers the situations in which violence has occurred before. This is often best done soon after a violent incident, so that possible triggers are more easily pinpointed.

One way of dealing with the possibility of impending violence is simple avoidance — encourage the relative to keep out of the patient's way, go to another room, or out of the house. Identifiable topics or situations that tend to make the patient angry should be avoided if possible. The strategy of avoidance can be quite effective, but it has the drawback that nothing in the situation is changed, especially as it is not usually possible to keep the avoidance up for ever. One relative had learnt to recognize when tension was building up in her son from the expression on his face. When this happened, she would keep quiet and leave the room. However it was not always possible for her to stay out of the living room.

A somewhat more subtle policy is of deflection: if the patient seems to be experiencing a build-up of tension it may be possible to defuse it by suggesting some simple routine activity, going to the shops or doing some household chore. This obviously requires sensitivity and good judgement on the carer's part, as the wrong choice may make the situation worse. Sometimes relatives learn by experience that certain phrases are calming, and can be used to defuse the situation. One family would say 'why don't you go and have a lie down'. Sometimes this would work, but at other times, the suggestion would be received angrily. It then worked better to say 'well go out and buy me some cigarettes — here's the money — and come back when you feel calmer'.

A more direct approach is for staff and carers to confront the patient. This must not be done angrily of course, but in a neutral way that enables the patient to express angry feelings in a controlled setting. The aim must be to enable the expression of angry feeling without the patient having to act on them. Providing a forum where disagreements can be aired without leading to violence will help to defuse them. Even if patients and carers cannot alter their behaviour much at home, it may help to know that difficulties can be discussed at the next session, and a violent scene may thus be averted.

Sometimes the patient may become violent because they have misinterpreted things. This may be the sort of misinterpretation that anyone can make, but which those who are upset and distressed may make more easily, or it can be the result of delusional ideas. In either case, if carers realize that the patient is becoming angry because of misinterpretation, they may be able to clarify the situation by gentle questioning. If the misinterpretation is not a delusional one, it may be possible for them to clear things up. If it is delusional, it may help to draw lines between the patients' reality and the carers', in the manner suggested on p. 132. However far the relative can get with clarifying misinterpretations, it is important for them to keep the transaction quiet and calm, using a firm and unflustered voice. If they can give the impression that they are not going to become upset or angry, this gives the patient the feeling that things are under control, and this in turn will exert a calming influence. On some days, one patient would keep bursting in on her mother shouting threateningly 'I know you're trying to kill me, why are you making me feel ill'. Her mother had learnt that one response that would calm her down was to say firmly but clearly, 'no, I was just sitting here reading the paper. Please don't shout'. It was often helpful to use distraction as well: 'Why don't we go out for a walk/make a cup of tea'. Again such strategies can be suggested to families, and possibly modelled in a family session.

Very often violence is a response to frustration — it arises when carers feel they must refuse something the patient wants. This may happen sometimes anyway, but it is more likely if the ground rules of the relationship have not been made very clear. If relatives appear to have been inconsistent about what they regard as acceptable, violence may be the method the patient uses to get them to permit what they would really rather refuse. This underlines once more the importance of firmness and clarity in the carer/patient relationship. Even if patients are quite disturbed, they will still be able to recognize this firmness and realize that there are limits beyond which they cannot pass. Knowing where they stand in this way may actually help them feel safer. Firmness in this sense is not to be confused with bossiness or intrusiveness. 'We agreed how much money you should have each day. I can't give you any more', said with conviction, confidently and consistently when the previously agreed limit has been reached is one example of the right sort of firmness.

However, while consistency may be an ideal, it is not all that easy to achieve, particularly if the situation has been going on for a long time, and carers have not in the past been able to get help and guidance. If there has been inconsistency in the past, the pattern may sadly be impossible to modify. Inconsistency in one family member going hand in hand with violence in the other is a frequent cause of family break-up, although the relationship may stagger painfully on for a long time before this eventually happens. Usually when there is a break-up, the well relative feels extremely guilty, even though the decision was the only realistic and practicable one to take. The relationship in our experience which most frequently gets locked into violence in this way is that between a mother, often elderly, and her ill but vigorous son: however, it can happen in most types of relationship, and we know of caring husbands who have been at their wits' end and indeed intimidated by their wives' violence.

As staff we are aware that even carers who are quite skillful at managing their relationship with their mentally ill relative may still find that there are times when violent situations develop. It may not be possible to be completely in control of the situation all the time. After all, professional staff are hit and hurt by patients from time to time, and it may become a question of just being in the wrong place at the wrong time. It may help to point this out to carers, and to use this as a basis for considering the idea of damage limitation.

How can carers deal with the immediate threat or the fact of violence? It is of benefit if staff have helped carers and patients think out beforehand what might happen, and what they are prepared to do. It obviously depends to a major extent on how able they are to withstand an assault physically. The first principle is that immediately carers become aware that they might be attacked, they should avoid getting stuck in the corner of the room. They should try and keep the furniture between themselves and the patient, and leave the room if necessary and if possible. If they cannot get out, they may as a last resort have to use a chair or a blanket or jacket as a defence. They may need to leave the house and call or phone for help. It may help if they have made an arrangement with a neighbour or with staff beforehand. They should not be afraid to call the police if necessary.

Although the police may not be able to do very much before violence has actually occurred, they will often at least appear on the scene, and having several police officers around will frequently calm things down, even to the extent that, when they leave, the patient does not become so angry again. This matter of calling the police does require judgement — if carers get to the stage where the patient is continually having outbursts of rage and violence and the police are being called in repeatedly, this is no proper basis for a relationship. If the circumstances cannot be changed for the better, carers and patients may then seriously have to consider parting company.

Sometimes there may be no escape or possibility of help, and the threat of violence may be so immediate and dangerous that carers have to comply with things against their will. This is particularly the case if patients have knives or guns, but also applies if they are much bigger and stronger than the relative.

If patients have actually been violent towards carers, it is important to try and deal with it afterwards in a way that may reduce its recurrence. It is relatively unusual to be badly hurt by a mentally ill relative. Being hit is, however, often very upsetting even when the physical damage is slight, because it says something to carers about the relationship, and also about the future — that it may be unpleasant, violent, and uncontrollable.

It may be very difficult indeed for carers to deal with the aftermath of violence in a constructive way without the assistance of staff, and it is usually reasonable to arrange an urgent meeting of carer, patient and staff member. It is important that carers should gently but firmly confront patients with the fact that they have been violent and have upset those around them. This should be done later, when they have had time to settle down — perhaps the next day. Most acts of violence occur in the evening or at night time, and talking about it during daylight has a normalizing effect. It should be pointed out that carers were hurt and upset by the patients' behaviour — they may not realize the effect it has had. An attempt should then be made to get them to apologise — this emphasizes to them that they have gone beyond acceptable limits. At the same time the incident should be explored and an attempt made to find out why it happened. Patients may have been angry because they were frightened, rationally or otherwise, and reassurance may be very helpful. They may also have felt that carers were being unreasonable in some way. It may be possible to explain the situation and carers' views of it to them in a way that is reassuring. It may then be possible to resolve differences.

Finally, acts of violence often mean that the patient is relapsing, so relatives should be encouraged to alert staff to this so that further action may be considered.

Helping Relatives to Cope with Depressed Patients

If depressed mood is a significant problem, staff members should see carers for two main reasons. First, relatives are usually in a position to offer reassurance and practical support to patients. Secondly, they may be unsure of the best ways of doing this.

Many relatives find it very hard to maintain their relationship with patients who are depressed. It can be particularly exasperating for them to see their best efforts come to nought, and it is not surprising that many give up the attempt, and withdraw, emotionally at any rate. This naturally reinforces the sufferers' sense of guilt and poor opinion of themselves. It may not be possible to improve depressed mood radically, at least in the short-term, but there are things relatives can do that may lighten patients' suffering and ease their own sense of burden.

It should also be pointed out that although reassurance is important to depressed people, it must not be done in a crude way. Staff must make clear for instance that it is not reassuring for people to have their fears and worries dismissed. Relatives need to know that it is much better to listen to the basis of the worries, to take them seriously, to spot where patients are being unrealistic or oversensitive, and to put forward an alternative view. In the process their interest and concern will also help to enhance the patients' sense of self esteem.

When patients are depressed, relatives often feel they ought to try and take them out of themselves. To this end they may suggest various social activities, even a holiday. Staff should be wary of encouraging what is often a bad idea. If patients do not enjoy the occasion, the depression is likely to get worse. They will also feel guilty because they have spoilt things for others. Any social activity must therefore be carefully planned in the light of the sufferers' state of mind. Simple visits by relatives or close friends may be all patients can take, and as much as they can benefit from.

Even if depression is a persistent and significant part of patients' mental illness, there are still things relatives can be encouraged to do in order to help them. Indeed it should be pointed out to them how important it is that they are not seen to give up in their attempts. Relatives often find depressed people rather unrewarding to be with, and there is always a temptation for them to withdraw. To a certain extent, staff may have to sanction this as relatives may need time on their own, just to keep going.

Relatives also find clinging and dependent behaviour quite difficult.

Depression may reach the point where patients cannot actually manage particular responsibilities any more. The clinician may be able to help relatives identify that this point has been reached. Carers may then have to take on these responsibilities themselves or organize others to do so. Staff should suggest that the relatives take charge and take over all household decisions without negotiation, until this acute stage has passed.

Relatives should be persuaded that even if they are doing most of the important things, they should still encourage patients to do something, even though it does not seem worth the trouble it causes them. When one patient became depressed his daughter would still get him to dry the dishes even though it was as much as he could manage. He could only do this very slowly and under close supervision, but she still thought it was important that he should do it. It gave her something to thank him for, and it allowed him the feeling of a task done.

Relatives sometimes get involved in long discussions about trivial matters that get nowhere because patients continually change the basis of the argument. Such disputes are pointless, and relatives should be advised to avoid them or at least try and defer them. Sometimes sufferers may become very opinionated about family matters, and this can also lead to long arguments that fail to produce constructive solutions.

In a minority of long-term patients depression may take the form of long lasting misery that seems unaffected by treatment. This is very difficult indeed to live with. Staff should be prepared to sanction relatives to protect themselves from the patients' misery at least for part of the time, by organizing their life away from them to an extent. This course of action will not do much to improve the patients' mood, but at least it may enable relatives to continue looking after them.

Threats of Suicide

In some long-term patients suicidal feelings and attempts may be a near-rational response to hopeless circumstances, but in other cases the cause is much less apparent. Staff should recall that sufferers may be most at risk when there has been some initial improvement. Not unnaturally, relatives feel panicked by the thought of suicide, and think that every opportunity must be blocked at all costs. This may lead to over-restrictive behaviour on their part that requires careful management by staff. Staff should aim to provide some sort of perspective on the risks and on appropriate responses. After all, it is not possible to prevent all suicide attempts, and determined individuals can often be successful, even when under apparently close surveillance.

Threats of suicide can be very upsetting and difficult to deal with. Some relatives may have the commonly held idea that people who talk frequently about suicide never actually try to kill themselves. They should be disabused of this, and persuaded that *all threats of suicide should be taken seriously*. It is difficult to communicate an appropriate attitude towards suicidal talk, and this must be done carefully in the light of the specific circumstances. While some of our patients sometimes make threats for effect or as a means of conveying distress, at other times they may be most seriously intent on killing themselves. Relatives and staff may both find it difficult to tell one kind of threat from another. Staff should advise relatives to take sensible precautions, such as not leaving tablets lying around the house and informing the hospital if patients seem more than normally tearful, morose or hopeless. Sometimes relatives may be unobservant about patients' moods. It can be helpful to talk through with them how the patient behaves when he or she is feeling down. The clinician can then suggest possible courses of action, simple things like getting relatives to ask patients how they are feeling; sometimes it suffices just to notice the sadness and attempt to offer comfort and reassurance if it will be accepted. It is worth pointing out that an arm round the shoulders or a cuddle may sometimes be easier than words, and often more effective.

Relatives of the long-term group of patients sometimes have to deal with actual attempts at suicide. Most such attempts these days involve self-poisoning. Relatives should be advised to seek medical help if there is *any possibility at all* that patients could have swallowed more than a usual dose of a drug, or that they retain an intention to end their life. At the same time it should be pointed out that some drugs like paracetomol (Panadol) can be fatal after a delay, even though they appear to have no immediate effects. The relative should be advised that, in any case of overdose, they should seek general medical, rather than psychiatric, help. If there is any suspicion that the overdose might be a dangerous one, they should either take the patient to a casualty department or phone 999 for an ambulance.

Effects on Sexual Relationships

Spouses of mentally ill people are often concerned about sexual aspects of their relationship. Many long-term patients lose much of their sexual desire and interest, sometimes as a result of medication. When combined with a loss of more general expressions of affection, this can be particularly difficult for partners to understand or accept. Improvement in the patients' condition may mean that sexual interest returns. Relatives may however find that their relationship has been changed, perhaps that their feelings have changed irrevocably, putting in doubt the continuation of the partnership. All the spouses we have talked to in this situation have wanted to end the relationship at one time or another, although the guilt this produces can be equally unbearable. Divorce is no longer uncommon in our society, and some relationships cannot accommodate a severe mental illness. Some couples however do find that such experiences draw them closer together than they have been before.

Partners may find these issues very difficult to talk about, and it may require delicate probing by staff before they will do so. Once clinicians have gained their confidence, partners may need considerable support in order to work through their complicated emotions. It is not the job of staff members to be judgemental over these issues, although this can be difficult to avoid as they will experience divided loyalties. The clinician's relationship with patients requires careful handling at this point as there is a danger that they will see support given to partners as a collusion against them. Maintaining fair and frank relationships with both patient and partner through this difficult period is crucial if staff are to salvage the best arrangement for the patient afterwards. Once relieved of the burden of a legal tie and an uninterrupted obligation to patients, relatives are sometimes able to offer more effective and less fraught support. The wife of one of our patients did divorce him some years back, and they no longer live together. However, she continues to be fond of him, and has him to stay some weekends and for most public holidays. She remains a major support, and the current arrangement seems to work much better than the marriage did.

Children in the Family

Relatives often worry that other members of the family, especially patients' children, will be adversely affected by the strain of living with someone suffering a severe mental illness. Staff should explore with them the possibility of getting help from neighbours, friends and other relatives. This may be crucial in relieving strains, and will mean that children have other adults to turn to if required. Staff should encourage relatives to give a reasonable and simple explanation even to younger children. Children are often given confusing messages about 'Daddy going away'. This usually makes them feel insecure and upset, perhaps that in some way it is their fault. Carers should be encouraged to talk to children in a period of calm about some of the experiences that their parents have when they are ill. The experiences can be compared to being in a dream, not necessarily a pleasant one, that continues even when their parent is awake. This can be used to explain why parents may be preoccupied or upset, or seem less caring or interested in the children. Staff should encourage carers to take the needs of older children equally seriously, as they can themselves often be supportive to carers and patients alike, provided they are given a chance to understand the problems, and difficulties are dealt with calmly so that upsetting or frightening crises are avoided. If problems do become too difficult for families with dependent children, the staff member can usually rely on back-up from the local social services department, health visitor, or child guidance clinic. Sometimes it may be necessary to make obligations statutory through the At Risk Register.

Occasionally problems in families where there are children may seem insurmountable. Staff members may then have to seek the help of the team social worker or the local authority social services department to arrange domestic help or a substitute carer on a temporary basis. In exceptional circumstances it may be necessary for staff to arrange for children to be placed temporarily in the care of the local authority with foster parents or in a children's home. This should only occur if there is no familiar alternative person, such as another relative or friend, who is able and suitable to care for them.

Another major worry that affects families is the possibility that children may inherit the tendency to the disorder. It pays staff members to know something of the risks, which are real but differ according to the exact circumstances. The worst situation is very unusual, and is when both parents have schizophrenia. In this case, around half of the children will be affected by the disease. Normally, only one parent has schizophrenia. Overall, the risk that a child with one affected and one unaffected parent will themselves develop schizophrenia is about 10%, but this varies, depending on a number of factors. It is less when the parent's schizophrenia is associated with a recognizable non-inherited cause, like birth injury, head injury or epilepsy. It is also less if no-one else in the family has the disease. The risk is greater when the parent's schizophrenia is of a severe type. The inherited risk for bipolar manic depressive disorder is probably about the same as for schizophrenia, that for unipolar disorder somewhat less.

The fact that these disorders are partly inherited raises the question of whether people who develop them should choose to have children if they have not already done so. Most professionals would feel that the genetic risk in the majority of cases is of a degree that should not necessarily deter possible parents. Obviously this is a decision that must be taken by the couple, and the genetic risk is actually a relatively minor consideration. Much more important is whether the illness seriously undermines the sufferer's ability to carry out the duties and everyday responsibilities of parenthood, and staff may have to talk this issue through at some length.

In some centres, staff members may be able to refer the carer to a Genetic Counselling Service. They should make it their business to know if there is one in the area.

Money Problems

Quite apart from the more extreme financial indiscretions seen in the active phase of mania, many patients may have to rely totally on social security or sickness benefit. They may find it impossible to budget, and demand extra money from relatives to pay for cigarettes, alcohol or daily necessities. The latter may find these demands difficult to refuse, but resent the fact patients cannot be more responsible or independent.

In circumstances like these, it may be worthwhile for staff to help carers to organize a daily budget for the patient, so that money is spaced out over the week and not spent all at once. Following suggestions from staff, one patient and her mother were able to agree that she should have £2 a day for herself. Clothing and other items were bought rarely, but were to come out of their joint money. Gradually, as she became better at managing, it was possible to phase out this daily allowance system.

Patients' spouses may find money problems particularly worrying. If the illness prevents the breadwinner from working, financial problems can indeed cause great hardship, particularly if there are young children. Sometimes it may be effective for staff to suggest that patients and partners change roles, so erstwhile breadwinners help more in the home while their partners go out to work. Because of entrenched views about what men and women ought to do, it is not always easy to persuade carers and patients that this is an appropriate course of action. Moreover, even simple household tasks will be too much for some patients, especially if they have recently suffered a relapse, and other friends and relatives may have to help with child care and housework.

Practical help with benefits may sometimes ease a financial burden. There may be other ways of taking some of the pressures off the family by helping it to maintain its income. Staff should be flexible in suggesting or organizing home helps, day nurseries or play groups, and occupation and leisure activities such as day centres, workshops or clubs.

If carers are worried because patients seem to be getting into difficulties in managing money or property, it may be appropriate for staff to suggest that patients take out a Power of Attorney authorizing carers or some other person to handle their property. This legal document depends on patients being able to understand what is meant by signing it, and if they become mentally incapable afterwards, the power is revoked. They themselves may also revoke it at any time. If patients are so mentally disordered that their power of attorney would be invalid, it might then be worth suggesting to carers that they apply to the *Court of Protection*. This will assess the medical evidence and may appoint a *Receiver*, who is likely to be the carer. He or she would then have control over the patient's property, and duties such as investing money, settling debts and keeping property in good repair. Unlike an ordinary Power of Attorney, patients cannot revoke this arrangement although they may submit objections to the Court if they do not agree to it.

Advising About the Use of Alcohol

Staff members may have problems over patients' use of alcohol, as there may be a conflict between the desirable and the possible. Most physicians recommend that anyone on psychotropic medication should drink very little alcohol, if indeed any. There are good reasons for this. The major tranquillizers cause an exaggeration of the normal effects of alcohol, and patients may quickly become sleepy, morose, or less in control of their emotions.

However, this may be quite unrealistic. Long-term patients may greatly resent being given rules about drinking, whether by professionals or by their relatives, and may rightly feel that alcohol is the only pleasure they now enjoy. Staff may also have to educate other members of the family about the effects of alcohol and the current thinking about how much is acceptable. In general, a couple of pints of beer or two or three glasses of wine every other day may have to be accepted. As a rule of thumb, staff should advise the family to think of medication as doubling the potency of alcohol, so the effect of a pint of beer is likely to equal that of two pints in former times. It may be that a little cautious experimentation is required. Patients vary considerably in their degree of control over alcohol consumption. Clinicians should try to foster calm discussion about alcohol consumption with the patient and other members of the family.

Some families, fortunately not a majority, find that difficulties over patients' alcohol consumption and their resulting behaviour can be one of the worst aspects of the illness. Sufferers may not actually drink to what would normally be regarded as excess, but because even small amounts of alcohol can have effects when combined with drugs, the results of quite moderate drinking can be very unpleasant. One man who lived with his mother would nag and worry her every night for money for a few beers. She would give in to him against her better judgement and he would go to the pub, returning home drunk to be sick over the bed. It took considerable negotiation between the patient, his mother and the hospital staff before this pattern was changed, and he was able to behave in a more acceptable manner.

Staff were able to suggest a successful strategy to another patient's mother. When he said he wanted a bottle of whisky, she would agree that they both needed a drink and offer to buy one on her next shopping trip. She would do this, and for a few nights afterwards, they had a couple of drinks together. After that the patient lost interest, and the bottle remained half full in the cupboard.

Problems with Medication

Ideally medication should be an arrangement between staff and patients, and in many cases there is no problem about this. Nevertheless, failure to comply with medication is one of the most frequent reasons for deterioration in those suffering from longstanding mental illness. For this reason, it may be appropriate for staff to liaise with carers over this issue. At the simplest level, it is important to remove carers' misapprehensions about the role of medication, as this will at least ensure they do not insidiously sabotage the patients' compliance.

It may take considerable staff time to get across just why medication is being prescribed. The rationale in the long-term group is of course largely prophylactic and we have found that this is a particularly difficult concept to communicate. It is sometimes (but not always!) useful to provide an analogy; for instance, with the use of insulin in diabetes.

There are several specific ways in which carers can assist with medication. Involvement may need only to be minimal: relatives should provide support and encouragement for patients in taking medication, acknowledging to them how difficult it can be to have to take drugs for extended periods. Sometimes a little more is needed, and relatives can provide occasional verbal prompting to patients, thereby reminding them to take the medication regularly. Occasionally patients simply forget to take their medication. If they do this regularly, it is useful for staff members, carers and patients to discuss how a routine can be established — relatively simple techniques often work, such as getting the patient into the habit of putting a tablet out at meal times.

If relatively low key and unobtrusive techniques like this prove unsuccessful, it often means that someone has to take over responsibility for ensuring compliance. This need not be the relative; it can be done by having the patient receive their drugs at the day hospital. The advantage of this is that it prevents medication becoming a focus of argument for the family. If the relatives do take over responsibility for giving the patient tablets at the prescribed times, this really has to be done with the patient's acceptance.

Even if relatives are not supervising medication it can be useful to get them to report back to staff if they suspect tablets are being left in the bottle or put down the toilet. Again this works best if it is agreed in principle beforehand between staff, patient and relative. Otherwise it has connotations of spying, and many patients are sensitive enough to such ideas without having additional provocations.

Finally, if none of these strategies work, staff may have to consider a change in regime, perhaps to an injectable form of medication. This is not always easy to manage as patients may understandably find injections aversive.

Helping Carers to Recognize Relapse

In most cases, particularly if relapse has occurred before, relatives will be the best judge of whether patients are becoming ill again. However, it is often useful to set time aside in order to discuss possible signs of relapse with them. The relatives may learn something, and so indeed may the clinician.

The early stages of relapse may be subtle and pose a real problem for carers. On one hand, if they can recognize a relapse early, it can probably be preempted by prompt treatment. On the other, it makes the relationship difficult if they are always on the alert for signs of relapse, and everything patients do is evaluated to see if it is normal or might be the effect of illness. Obviously a balance has to be struck, and staff members should aim to help carers to reach this.

For example, increased irritability may be an early indicator of relapse, particularly in mania. This has to be judged against normal loss of temper, and relatives sometimes find it hard to distinguish between a normal response and an excessive one, given the particular circumstances. Although relatives are as likely to make this judgement correctly as staff members, it may still be useful to discuss the matter, and also to negotiate it with the patient.

The various behavioural changes associated with relapse in

schizophrenia include changes in sleep pattern and appetite, social withdrawal, deteriorating self-care, an increase in suspiciousness or a return to former preoccupations. Relapse may also be heralded by feelings of tenseness and nervousness, and it may be difficult for relatives to grasp that these indicate something more sinister.

The major changes may be of mood: patients may become increasingly nervous or depressed. However, people with schizophrenia sometimes become depressed without it indicating relapse: they often have enough to be depressed about, so again it may be hard for relatives to distinguish these reactions to their unrewarding situation from the symptoms of relapse. Relapse in severe affective disorder may be particularly difficult to spot because it is often so gradual.

Sometimes the form of the relapse may change, and this may make it difficult for relatives to identify it or even to acknowledge that it has happened. One of our patients with severe manic depressive illness usually became overactive and talkative when he relapsed. Recently a relapse took the form of irritability, and it required a lot of work by staff to persuade his parents that he had indeed experienced a further episode. This illustrates that clinicians may have to make a point of interpreting the symptoms of a particular breakdown to diminish potential misattribution by relatives.

Relapse in some patients is heralded by idiosyncratic behaviour, the significance of which would be lost on the uninitiated onlooker. It is often a good idea for staff to explore with relatives whether such signs exist for a given patient. So, for example, relatives may hear patients tossing and turning, or moving around the house at odd hours. When one patient was relapsing, she took over the task of walking the dog and began to make slightly unrealistic plans for a return to work. Another patient would frown when he experienced a return of delusional concerns. The identification of such idiosyncrasies help both staff and relatives to recognize impending relapse and to take avoiding action.

Dealing with Emergencies

Good care of long-term mentally ill patients should allow most episodes of deterioration to be picked up quickly and acted upon. Sometimes, however, patients deteriorate very rapidly, and relatives need to deal with urgent situations. However, they may not always know the best way of doing this. It is one of the clinician's tasks to anticipate problems of this type and to explore with relatives just what action they should take depending on the time and circumstances. Obviously, it is not possible for clinicians to foresee every possibility, but they should provide general guidelines for relatives. Staff members should put time aside at an opportune moment to do this. Sometimes it is appropriate to do this during a relatives' group. They need to be quite clear who the key worker is, and that they should contact him or her, or at the very least some other member of the team. They should also be told what to do out of hours; it may then be necessary to seek the help of the local psychiatric emergency clinic (if there is one!). If there is no emergency facility, relatives should be advised to go through the family doctor, and this is one reason for the team maintaining good relations with the primary care team.

Sometimes, relatively urgent situations arise when patients and their families are away from home. It is useful to advise them what to do if urgent action becomes necessary to deal with an emerging crisis. They may need to enlist the help of local, temporary, GPs, who in turn may arrange admission to a nearby hospital to start with. Patients can then be transferred to their own local hospital when it is convenient and practicable. Relatives should be advised that it is probably not a good idea to go to a general hospital casualty department with a purely psychiatric problem.

The relatives of most long-term patients know only too well the procedures surrounding compulsory admission. However, they may still be understandably reluctant to initiate actions that may lead to an admission of this type. Clinicians may have to work through this reluctance on the relatives' part, encouraging them to see that in certain circumstances it is a reasonable course of action that will be of benefit to the patient. If a very disturbed patient leaves the house and the relative is seriously worried, this may involve informing the local police. A good psychiatric team dealing with long-term patients should in any case foster relations with the local police station. Some of our relatives, living as they do in an inner city area, have attitudes towards the police that may not be entirely positive, and it is sometimes necessary for staff members to offer particular reassurance and support if they have had to enlist police assistance.

10 · Recapitulation

In this book we have based our suggestions for working with families on the research literature developed around the concept of Expressed Emotion. This is extensive and largely convincing. Although not all workers are happy with the ideas behind EE, we have found that it forms a useful framework. It has considerable clinical credibility, and is thus able to provide aims and formulations against which achievements can be evaluated. Because of this it can be used to foster optimism in staff and families.

The other important body of literature relevant to working with families is that concerning burden. The consistent finding of considerable burden has particular application to the relatives and carers of those with the more longstanding and severe mental illnesses. They carry out the caring role year in, year out, and many make a very impressive job of it, too. This may become uncomfortably apparent when for some reason they are no longer able to continue, whether because of exhaustion, infirmity or death. We have had experience of this: the loss of a carer often means that the clinical team has enormous difficulty in helping the patient maintain the same quality of life.

This literature, taken together, provides strong pragmatic grounds for involving carers as part of the clinical management of longstanding mental illness. This enables therapeutic resources to be maximized and may permit the planned generalization of skills into different settings. After all, patients usually spend more time where they live than in hospital facilities. In our view there is also a clear ethical obligation towards carers.

The *principles* involved in work of this kind can be summarized:

1 It requires *an open and frank relationship*. In establishing this relationship, the first priority is to be *sensitive to the needs* of the relatives. In our experience, the EE literature has alerted many clinicians to the important role of relatives, but in some cases this has had an untoward consequence, in that they are in too much of a hurry to evaluate the contribution of the

family situation to the course of the illness. While it is important to do this, clinicians will come badly unstuck if they start off with this as their primary target. Moreover, many have interpreted the literature to imply that only high EE relatives are in need of assistance. This is not true: many low EE relatives have problems, often relating to isolation, and the proper clinical approach in our view should primarily centre around the evaluation of problems. Assessing the influence of relatives on the patients' illness should be secondary to this.

2 *Positive attitudes* towards relatives and carers are crucial. Like all of us, they sometimes make mistakes; nevertheless clinicians should avoid the easy complacency of feeling that they could have done better in the circumstances. Most relatives do the best job they can over many years, in situations where the rewards are not obvious. The first task of clinicians in establishing relationships with carers is to engage in a process of *deliberate and active empathy*, to try and put themselves on the inside of the relatives' position. Sensitive appreciation of the carers' position will reveal the overlap with that of clinical staff, who face many of the same problems and require support and encouragement in the same way if they are to avoid burnout.

3 The *format* of intervention is probably not crucial, and should be decided in the light of local resources and preferences. In our view, no one model is best. Relevant considerations include the geographical characteristics of the health authority area, car ownership, and the convenience of staff and carers. In many settings relatives' groups are effective, provided they are energetically organized. Some families will always require individual sessions, and some will need to have them at home. Some are best served by a combination of relatives' groups and family sessions: as we pointed out in Chapter 4, these formats provide complementary advantages.

4 The *content* of intervention can be specified with some confidence. It is necessary for staff to offer *information*, to answer questions, and to share both knowledge and ignorance with the carers. Carers must be given time and space to *work through the emotional consequences* of their situation. It is also important to facilitate and improve *communication* by direct encouragement of listening skills and by modelling appropriate responses towards patients. Clinicians must evaluate the

effectiveness of relatives in *solving practical difficulties*: it will almost always be found appropriate to enhance the relatives' problem solving skills directly. The *scheduling* of these interventions demands considerable thought. Finally clinicians must be prepared to accept that *not all problems are soluble*, certainly in existing circumstances.

5 *Perspective* is crucial both to professionals and to carers. If professionals are looking to an unrealistically short-time span, their patient management will be badly planned. They will almost always be disappointed, with the consequence that motivation will be difficult to maintain. Moreover, relatives and carers almost always start off with the wrong perspective, and clinicians who themselves have unrealistic views of the likely schedule of progress will be in no position to help them over this.

6 The need to evaluate improvement over long stretches of time emphasizes another essential requirement for members of the staff team, namely, *persistence*. For improvement to happen at all, they must persevere in their attempts to achieve their chosen aims. This does not mean the stereotyped repetition of a single therapeutic approach, but the flexible deployment of strategies designed to attain long-term goals by one means or another. Circumstances, methods, and the identity of key personnel may change, but the team must organize itself so that one way or another it does not give up on the patients and families it is responsible for, even when some of the problems are insoluble. This aim may not be achieved, but is more likely to be approached if the operation of the team is designed to maintain morale and achieve continuity. The hard work and successes of team members must be readily, regularly and publicly acknowledged by their team colleagues, and they should be supported through the inevitable difficulties that arise in this sort of work.

7 Many patients have *very reduced social networks*, and this makes it likely that the people they do relate to are particularly important to them. In many cases, these will be family members, but sometimes other patients and members of staff in hostels, group homes and day centres come to be the most important people in the patients' lives. When this happens, it is worth being aware that these key persons take on many of the burdens of care, and have many of the same needs as relatives. Effective integration of the efforts of such people

into the overall management of patients maximizes resources and contains potential stresses in the same way as the involvement of relatives.

8 *Planning ahead* is a vital element of good long-term care. This may involve consideration of relatively remote eventualities, such as the death of a parent who is a carer, as described on p. 93. It should also be directed at the management of more immediate stresses that are known to be in the offing for patients whose mental state is fragile, such as a visit to relatives at some distance.

'It helps to realize that other people have to face similar problems, and that we are not alone' (relative of a long-term patient).

References

Al Khani M.A.F., Bebbington P.E., Watson J.P. et al. (1986). Life events and schizophrenia: a Saudi Arabian study. *British Journal of Psychiatry*, **148**, 12–22.

Anderson C.M., Hogarty G., Bayer T. et al. (1984). EE and social networks in parents of schizophrenic patients. *British Journal of Psychiatry*, **144**, 247–255.

Anderson C.M., Reiss D.J., Hogarty G.E. (1986). *Schizophrenia in the Family: A practitioner's guide to psychoeducation and management.* New York: Guilford Press.

Arieti S. (1959). Schizophrenia. In *The American Handbook of Psychiatry*, Vol. 1. (Arieti S. ed.). New York: Basic Books.

Barrelet L., Ferrero F., Szigetty L. et al. (1990). Expressed emotion and first admission schizophrenia: a replication in a French cultural environment. *British Journal of Psychiatry*, **156**, 357–362.

Barrowclough C., Tanier N., Watts S. et al. (1987). Assessing the functional value of relative's knowledge about schizophrenia: a preliminary report. *British Journal of Psychiatry*, **151**, 1–8.

Bateson G., Jackson D.D. Hally J. et al. (1956). Towards a theory of schizophrenia. *Behavioural Science*, **1**, 251–264.

Bebbington P.E. (1982). The course and prognosis of affective psychosis. In *Cambridge Handbook of Psychiatry*, Vol. III. (Wing J.K. ed.). Cambridge: Cambridge University Press.

Bebbington P.E. (1987). Life events and schizophrenia: The WHO collaborative study. *Social Psychiatry*, **22**, 179–180.

Bebbington P.E. (1988). Review of the Nithsdale Schizophrenia Survey VII. Does relatives' high Expressed Emotion predict relapse. *Transmissions*, **1**, 14–15.

Bebbington P.E., Kuipers L. (1988). Social influences on schizophrenia. In *Schizophrenia: The Major Issues*, (Bebbington P., McGuffin P. eds.). Oxford: Heinemann Medical.

Bebbington P.E., Kuipers L. (1991). Life events and social factors. In *Schizophrenia: an Interdisciplinary Handbook for Practitioners.* (Kavanagh D.J. ed.). London: Chapman & Hall.

Beels C.C. (1979). Social networks in schizophrenia. *Psychiatric Quarterly*, **51**, 209–215.

Belknap I. (1956). *Human Problems of a State Mental Hospital*, New York: McGraw-Hill.

Berkowitz R., Eberlein-Friess R., Kuipers, L. et al. (1984): Educating relatives about schizophrenia. *Schizophrenia Bulletin*, **10**, 418–429.

Birchwood M., Smith J. (1987). Schizophrenia in the family. In *Coping with Disorder in the Family*. (Orford J. ed.). London: Croom Helm.

Birtchnell J., Kennard J. (1983). Does marital maladjustment lead to mental illness? *Social Psychiatry*, **18**, 79–88.

Bledin K., MacCarthy B., Kuipers L. et al. (1990). EE in the daughters of the demented elderly. *British Journal of Psychiatry* (in press).

Brown G.W. (1959). Experiences of discharged chronic schizophrenic mental hospital patients in various types of living group. *Millbank Memorial Fund Quarterly*, **37**, 105–131.

Brown G.W. (1974). Meaning, measurement and stress of life events. In *Stressful Life Events: Their Nature and Effects*. (Dohrenwend B.S., Dohrenwend B.P. eds.). New York: John Wiley.

Brown G.W., Carstairs G.M., Topping G.C. (1958). The post hospital adjustment of chronic mental patients. *Lancet*, **ii**, 685–689.

Brown G.W., Monck E.M., Carstairs G.M. et al. (1962). Influence of family life on the course of schizophrenic illness. *British Journal of Preventive and Social Medicine*, **16**, 55–68.

Brown G., Bone M., Dalison B. et al. (1966). *Schizophrenia and Social Care*. Oxford: Oxford University Press.

Brown G.W., Rutter M.L. (1966). The measurement of family activities and relationships. *Human Relations*, **19**, 241–263.

Brown G.W., Birley J.L.T. (1968). Crises and life changes and the onset of schizophrenia. *Journal of Health and Social Behaviour*, **9**, 203–214.

Brown G.W., Birley J.L.T., Wing, J.K. (1972). Influence of family life on the course of schizophrenic disorders: A replication. *British Journal of Psychiatry*, **121**, 241–258.

Brown G.W., Harris T.O., Peto J. (1973). Life events and psychiatric disorders. Part 2: Nature of causal link. *Psychological Medicine*, **3**, 159–176.

Brown G.W., Harris T.O. (1978). *Social Origins of Depression*. London: Tavistock.

Budzyna-Dawidowski P., Rostworowska M., de Barbaro B. (1989). Stability of Expressed Emotion. A 3 year follow-up study of schizophrenic patients. Paper presented at the 19th Annual Congress of the European Association of Behaviour Therapy, Vienna, Sept 10–24.

Canton G., Fraccon I.G. (1985). Life events and schizophrenia: a replication. *Acta Psychiatrica Scandinavica*, **71**, 211–216.

Cazzullo C.L., Bertrando P., Bressi C. et al. (1989). Expressed Emotion in Italian families: A comparison between schizophrenics and other patients. Paper resented at the 19th Annual Congress of the European Association of Behaviour Therapy, Vienna, Sept 20–24.

Clausen J.A., Yarrow M.R. (1955a). The impact of mental illness on the family. *Journal of Social Issues*, **11**, 3–64.

Clausen J.A., Yarrow M.R., Deasy L.C. et al. (1955b). The impact of mental illness: research formulation. *Journal of Social Issues*, **11**, 6–11.

Collins J., Kreitman N., Nelson B. et al. (1971). Neurosis and marital interaction: III Family roles and functions. *British Journal of Psychiatry*, **119**, 233–242.

Cozolino L.J., Goldstein M.J., Nuechterlein K.S. et al. (1988). The impact of education about schizophrenia on relatives varying in levels of Expressed Emotion. *Schizophrenia Bulletin*, **14**, 675–686.

Creer C., Wing J.K. (1974). *Schizophrenia at Home*. Surbiton, National Schizophrenia Fellowship.

Creer C., Wing J.K. (1975). Living with a schizophrenic patient. *British Journal of Hospital Medicine*, **14**, 73–82.

Creer C., Sturt E., Wykes T. (1982). The role of relatives. In: Long term community care: experience in a London borough (Wing J.K. ed.) pp. 29–39. *Psychological Medicine*, Monograph, Supplement 2.

Crow T.J. (1989). A current view of the Type II syndrome: age of onset, intellectual impairment and the meaning of structural changes in the brain. *British Journal of Psychiatry*, **155** (suppl 7), 10–14.

Day R. (1986). Social stress and schizophrenia: from the concept of recent life events to the notion of toxic environments. In *Handbook of Studies on Schizophrenia*, (Burrows G.D., Norman T.R. eds.). Amsterdam: Elsevier.

Day R., Neilsen J.A., Korten A. et al. (1987). Stressful life events preceding the acute onset of schizophrenia: a cross-national study from the World Health Organization. *Culture, Medicine and Psychiatry*, **11**, 123–206.

Deasy L.C., Quinn O.W. (1955). The wife of the mental patient and the hospital psychiatrist. *Journal of Social Issues*, **11**, 49–60.

Doane J.A., West K.L., Goldstein M.J. et al. (1981). Parental communication deviance and affective style: predictors of subsequent schizophrenia spectrum disorders in vulnerable adolescents. *Archives of General Psychiatry*, **38**, 679–685.

Doane J.A., Falloon I.R.H., Goldstein M.J. et al. (1985). Parental affective style and the treatment of schizophrenia: predicting course of illness and social functioning. *Archives of General Psychiatry*, **42**, 34–42.

Doane J.A., Goldstein M.J., Miklowitz D.J. et al. (1986). The impact of individual and family treatment on the affective climate of families of schizophrenia. *British Journal of Psychiatry*, **148**, 279–287.

Dulz B., Hand I. (1986). Short term relapse in young schizophrenics: Can it be predicted and affected by family (CFI), patient, and treatment variables? An experimental study. In *Treatment of Schizophrenia: Family Assessment and Intervention*. (Goldstein, M.J., Hand I., Hahlweg

K. eds.). Berlin: Springer.

Dunham H.W., Weinberg S.K. (1960). *Culture of the State Mental Hospital*, Detroit: Wayne State University Press.

Fadden G.B., Bebbington P.E., Kuipers L. (1987a). The burden of care: the impact of functional psychiatric illness on the patient's family. *British Journal of Psychiatry*, **150**, 285–292.

Fadden G.B., Kuipers L., Bebbington P.E. (1987b). Caring and its burdens: a study of the relatives of depressed patients. *British Journal of Psychiatry*, **151**, 660–667.

Falloon I.R.H., Boyd J.L., McGill C.W. et al. (1982). Family management in the prevention of exacerbations of schizophrenia. A controlled study. *New England Journal of Medicine*, **306**, 1437–1440.

Falloon I.R.H., Boyd J.L., McGill C.W. (1984). *Family Care of Schizophrenia*. New York: Guilford Press.

Falloon I.R.H., Boyd J.L., McGill C.W. et al. (1985). Family management in the prevention of morbidity of schizophrenia. Clinical outcome of a two year longitudinal study. *Archives of General Psychiatry*, **42**, 887–896.

Falloon I.R.H., Pederson J. (1985). Family management in the prevention of morbidity of schizophrenia. Adjustment of the family unit. *British Journal of Psychiatry*, **147**, 156–163.

Favre S., Gonzales C., Lendais G. et al. (1989). Expressed Emotion (EE) of schizophrenic relatives. Poster presented at VIIIth World Congress of Psychiatry, Athens, 12th–19th October.

Ferrera J.A., Vizarro C. (1989). Expressed Emotion and course of schizophrenia in a Spanish sample. Paper presented at the 19th Annual Congress of the European Association of Behaviour Therapy. Vienna, Sept 20–24.

Gantt A.B., Goldstein G., Pinky S. (1989). Family understanding of psychiatric illness. *Community Mental Health Journal*, **25**, 101–108.

Goffman E. (1961). *Asylums*, Harmondsworth, Penguin.

Goldberg S.C., Schooler N.R., Hogarty G.E. et al. (1977). Prediction of relapse in schizophrenic outpatients treated by drug and sociotherapy. *Archives of General Psychiatry*, **34**, 171–184.

Goldstein M. (1985). Family factors that antedate the onset of schizophrenia and related disorders: the results of a 15 year prospective longitudinal study. *Acta Psychiatrica Scandinavica*, **71**, Suppl 319, 7–18.

Goldstein M. (1987). The UCLA High-risk project. *Schizophrenia Bulletin*, **13**, 505–514.

Goldstein M., Judd L.L., Rodnick E.H., et al. (1968). A method for studying social influence and coping patterns within families of disturbed adolescents. *Journal of Nervous and Mental Disease*, **147**, 233–251.

Goldstein M., Strachan A. (1986). The impact of family intervention programmes on family communication and the short term course of schizophrenia. In *Treatment of Schizophrenia: Family Assessment and Intervention*. (Goldstein M.J., Hand I., Hahlweg K. eds.). Berlin: Springer.

Grad J., Sainsbury P. (1963a). Evaluating a community care service. In *Trends in Mental Health Services*. (Freeman H., Farndale J. eds.) pp. 303–317. New York: MacMillan Company.

Grad J., Sainsbury P. (1963b). Mental illness and the family. *Lancet*, **i**, 544–547.

Greedharry (1987). Expressed Emotion in the families of the mentally handicapped: A pilot study. *British Journal of Psychiatry*, **150**, 400–402.

Greenley J.R. (1986). Social control and Expressed Emotion. *Journal of Nervous and Mental Disease*, **174**, 24–30.

Haley J. (1976). *Problem Solving Therapy*. San Francisco. Jossey Bass.

Hemsley D.R. (1987). Psychological models of schizophrenia. In *Textbook of Abnormal Psychology*, (Miller E., Cooper P. eds.). Edinburgh: Churchill Livingstone.

Henderson S. (1980). Personal networks and the schizophrenias. *Australian and New Zealand Journal of Psychiatry*, **14**, 255–259.

Hewitt S., Ryan P., Wing J.K. (1975). Living without the mental hospitals. *Journal of Social Policy*, **4**, 391–404.

Hinchcliffe M.K., Hooper D., Roberts F.J. (1978). *The Melancholy Marriage*. Chichester: J. Wiley & Sons.

Hirsch S.R., Leff J.P. (1975). *Abnormalities in the Parents of Schizophrenics*. Maudsley Monograph No. 22. Oxford: Oxford University Press.

Hoenig J., Hamilton M.W. (1966). The schizophrenic patient in the community and his effect on the household. *International Journal of Social Psychiatry*, **12**, 165–176.

Hoenig J., Hamilton M.W. (1969). *The Desegregation of the Mentally Ill*. London, Routledge and Kegan Paul.

Hogarty G.E. (1985). Expressed Emotion and schizophrenic relapse: implications from the Pittsburg Study. In *Controversies in Schizophrenia*, (Alpert M. ed.). New York: Guilford Press.

Hogarty G.E., Anderson C.M., Reiss D.J. et al. (1986). Family psychoeducation, social skills training and maintenance chemotherapy in the aftercare treatment of schizophrenia. I. One year effects of a controlled study on relapse and Expressed Emotion. *Archives of General Psychiatry*, **43**, 633–642.

Hooley J.M. (1985). Expressed Emotion: a review of the critical literature. *Clinical Psychology Review*, **5**, 119–139.

Hooley J.M., Hahlweg K. (1986). The marriages and interaction patterns of depressed patients and their spouses: Comparison of high and low EE dyads. In *Treatment of Schizophrenia: Family Assessment and Intervention*. (Goldstein M.J., Hand I., Hahlweg K. eds.). Berlin: Springer.

Hooley J.M., Orley J., Teasdale J. (1986). Levels of Expressed Emotion and relapse in depressed patients. *British Journal of Psychiatry*, **148**, 642–647.

Hubschmid T., Zemp M. (1989). Interactions in high- and low-EE families. *Social Psychiatry and Psychiatric Epidemiology*, **24**, 113–119.

Hume C., Pullen I. (1986). *Rehabilitation in Psychiatry*. Edinburgh: Churchill Livingstone.

Ivanovic M., Vuletic Z. (1989). Expressed Emotion in the families of patients with a frequent type of schizophrenia and its influence on the course of illness. Paper presented at the 19th Annual Congress of the European Association of Behaviour Therapy. Vienna, Sept 20–24.

Jackson S.E., Schwab R.L., Schiller R.S. (1986). Towards an understanding of the Burnout Phenomenon. *Journal of Applied Psychology*, **71**, 630–640.

Jacobs S., Myers J. (1976). Recent life events and acute schizophrenic psychosis: a controlled study. *Journal of Nervous and Mental Disease*, **162**, 75–87.

Karno M., Jenkins J.H., de la Selva A. et al. (1987). Expressed Emotion and schizophrenic outcome among Mexican-American families. *Journal of Nervous and Mental Disease*, **175**, 143–151.

Kiloh L.G., Andrews G., Neilson M. (1988). The long-term outcome of depressive illness. *British Journal of Psychiatry*, **153**, 752–775.

Koenigsberg H.W., Handley R. (1986). Expressed Emotion: From predictive index to clinical construct. *American Journal of Psychiatry*, **143**, 1361–1373.

Köttgen C., Sonnichsen I., Mollenhauer K. et al. (1984). Group therapy with the families of schizophrenic patients: results of the Hamburg Camberwell Family Interview Study III. *International Journal of Family Psychiatry*, **5**, 84–94.

Kreisman D.E., Joy V.D. (1974). Family response to the mental illness of a relative: a review of the literature. *Schizophrenia Bulletin*, **10**, 34–57.

Kreitman N. (1964). The patient's spouse. *British Journal of Psychiatry*, **110**, 159–173.

Kreitman N., Collins J., Nelson B. et al. (1970). Neurosis and marital interaction: I Personality and symptoms. *British Journal of Psychiatry*, **117**, 33–46.

Kuipers L. (1979). Expressed Emotion: a review. *British Journal of Social and Clinical Psychology*, **18**, 237–243.

Kuipers L. (1983). Family factors in schizophrenia: an intervention study. Ph.D. Thesis. University of London.

Kuipers L. (1987). Depression and the family. In *Coping with Disorder in the Family*. (Orford J. ed.). London: Croom-Helm.

Kuipers L., Sturgeon D., Berkowitz R. et al. (1983). Characteristics of

Expressed Emotion: its relationship to speech and looking in schizophrenic patients and their relatives. *British Journal of Clinical Psychology*, **22**, 257–264.

Kuipers L., Bebbington P.E. (1985). Relatives as a resource in the management of functional illness. *British Journal of Psychiatry*, **147**, 465–471.

Kuipers L., Bebbington P.E. (1987). *Living with Mental Illness*. London: Souvenir Press.

Kuipers L., Bebbington P.E. (1988). Expressed Emotion research in schizophrenia: theoretical and clinical implications. *Psychological Medicine*, **18**, 893–910.

Kuipers L., MacCarthy B., Hurry J. et al. (1989). Counselling the relatives of the long term mentally ill. II. A low-cost supportive model. *British Journal of Psychiatry*, **154**, 775–782.

Laing R.D., Esterson A. (1964). *Sanity, Madness and the Family*, Harmondsworth, Penguin.

Lamb H.R. (1982). *Treating the Long-term Mentally Ill*. San Francisco, Jossey Bass.

Lee A.S., Murray R.M. (1988). The long-term outcome of Maudsley depressives. *British Journal of Psychiatry*, **153**, 741–751.

Leff J.P., Wing J.K. (1971). Trial of maintenance therapy in schizophrenia. *British Medical Journal*, **iii**, 599–604.

Leff J.P., Brown G.W. (1977). Family and social factors in the course of schizophrenia (letter). *British Journal of Psychiatry*, **130**, 417–420.

Leff J.P., Vaughn C.E. (1981). The role of maintenance therapy and relatives' Expressed Emotion in relapse of schizophrenia: a two year follow up. *British Journal of Psychiatry*, **139**, 102–104.

Leff J.P., Kuipers L., Berkowitz R. et al. (1982). A controlled trial of social intervention in schizophrenic families. *British Journal of Psychiatry*, **141**, 121–134.

Leff J.P., Kuipers L., Berkowitz R. et al. (1983). Life events, relatives' Expressed Emotion and maintenance neuroleptics in schizophrenic relapse. *Psychological Medicine*, **13**, 799–806.

Leff J.P., Kuipers L., Berkowitz R. et al. (1985). A controlled trial of social intervention in the families of schizophrenic patients: two year follow up. *British Journal of Psychiatry*, **146**, 594–600.

Leff J.P., Vaughn C. (1985). *Expressed Emotion in Families*. New York: The Guilford Press.

Leff J.P., Wig N., Ghosh A., et al. (1987). Influence of relatives' Expressed Emotion on the course of schizophrenia in Chandigarh. *British Journal of Psychiatry*, **151**, 166–173.

Leff J.P., Berkowitz R., Eberlein-Fries R. et al. (1988). *Schizophrenia: Notes for Relatives and Friends*. Surbiton, National Schizophrenia Fellowship.

Leff J., Berkowitz R., Sharit N. et al. (1989). A trial of family therapy v. a relatives' group for schizophrenia. *British Journal of Psychiatry*, **154**, 58–66.

Liberman R.P. (1986). Coping and competence as protective factors in the vulnerability – stress model of schizophrenia. In *Treatment of Schizophrenia: Family assessment and Intervention* (Goldstein M.J., Hand I., Hallweg K. eds.). 201–216. Berlin: Springer Verlag.

Liberman R.P., Jacobs H.E., Boon S.E. et al. (1987). Skills training for the community adaptation of schizophrenia. In *Psychosocial Treatment of Schizophrenia*. (Strauss J.S., Boker W., Brenner H.D. eds.). Toronto: Hans Huber.

Lidz T., Cornelison A.R., Fleck S. et al. (1957). The intrafamilial environment of the schizophrenic patient. I. *Psychiatry*, **20**, 329–342.

MacCarthy B., Hemsley D., Schrank-Fernandez C. et al. (1986). Unpredictability as a correlate of Expressed Emotion in the relatives of schizophrenics. *British Journal of Psychiatry*, **148**, 727–730.

MacCarthy B., Kuipers L., Hurry J. et al. (1989). Counselling the relatives of the long term mentally ill. I. Evaluation. *British Journal of Psychiatry*, **154**, 768–775.

MacCarthy B., Lesage A., Brewin C.R. et al. (1990). Needs for care among the relatives of long term users of day care. (In press).

McCreadie R.G., Robinson A.T.D. (1987). The Nithsdale Schizophrenia Survey: VI. Relatives' Expressed Emotion: prevalence, patterns and clinical assessment. *British Journal of Psychiatry*, **150**, 640–644.

McCreadie R.G., Phillips K. (1988). The Nithsdale Schizophrenia Survey: VII. Does relatives' high Expressed Emotion predict relapse? *British Journal of Psychiatry*, **152**, 477–481.

McCreadie R.G., Phillips K., Harvey J.A. et al. (1990). The Nithsdale Schizophrenia Surveys VIII. Do relatives want family intervention and does it help? *British Journal of Psychiatry*, (in press).

MacMillan J.F., Gold A., Crow T.J. et al. (1986). The Northwick Park Study of First Episodes of Schizophrenia. IV. Expressed Emotion and relapse. *British Journal of Psychiatry*, **148**, 133–143.

MacMillan J.F., Crow T.J., Johnson A.L. et al. (1987). Expressed Emotion and relapse in first episodes of schizophrenia. *British Journal of Psychiatry*, **151**, 320–323.

Malzacher M., Merz J., Ebnother D. (1981). Einschneidende Lebensereignisse im Vorfeld akuter schizophrener Episoden: Erstmals erkrankte Patienten im Vergleich mit einer Normalstichprobe. *Archiv für Psychiatrie und Nervenkrankheiten*, **230**, 227–242.

Mandelbrote B.M., Folkard S. (1961a). Some problems and needs of schizophrenics in relation to a developing psychiatric community service. *Comprehensive Psychiatry*, **2**, 317–328.

Mandelbrote B.M., Folkard S. (1961b). Some factors related to outcome and social adjustment in schizophrenia. *Acta Psychiatrica Scandinavica*, **37**, 223–235.

Mann S., Cree W. (1975). The 'new long-stay' in mental hospitals. *British Journal of Hospital Medicine*, **14**, 56–63.

Mavreas V., Tomaros V., Carydi N. et al. (1990). Expressed Emotion in families of chronic schizophrenics and its association with clinical measures (to be submitted).

Miklowitz D.J., Goldstein M.J., Falloon R.H. (1983). Premorbid and symptomatic characteristics of schizophrenics from families with high and low levels of Expressed Emotion. *Journal of Abnormal Psychology*, **92**, 359–367.

Miklowitz D.J., Goldstein M.J., Falloon R.H. et al. (1984). Interactional correlates of Expressed Emotion in the families of schizophrenics. *British Journal of Psychiatry*, **144**, 482–487.

Miklowitz D.J., Goldstein M.J., Nuechterlein K.H. et al. (1988). Family factors and the course of bipolar affective disorder. *Archives of General Psychiatry*, **45**, 225–231.

Miklowitz D.J., Goldstein M.J., Doane J.A. et al. (1989). Is Expressed Emotion an index of a transactional process. I. Parent's Affective Style. *Family Process*, **28**, 153–167.

Mills E. (1962). *Living with Mental Illness: A Study in East London*. London: Routledge and Kegan Paul.

Minuchin S. (1974). *Families and Family Therapy*. Cambridge Mass.: Harvard University Press.

Moline R.A., Singh S., Morris A. et al. (1985). Family Expressed Emotion and relapse in schizophrenia in 24 urban American patients. *American Journal of Psychiatry*, **142**, 1078–1081.

Mozny P. (1989). Expressed Emotion and rehospitalization rates of schizophrenics in the psychiatric hospital Kromeriz, CSSR. Paper presented at the 19th Annual Congress of the European Association of Behaviour Therapy, Vienna, Sept 20–24.

Nelson B., Collins J., Kreitman N. et al. (1970). Neurosis and marital interaction: II Time sharing and social activity. *British Journal of Psychiatry*, **117**, 47–58.

Nuechterlein K.H., Snyder K.S., Dawson M.E. et al, (1986). Expressed Emotion, fixed-dose fluphenazine decanoate maintenance, and relapse in recent onset schizophrenia. *Psychopharmacology Bulletin*, **22**, 633–639.

Orford J. (1986). *Coping with Disorder in the Family*. Croom-Helm.

Ovenstone I.M.K. (1973a). The development of neurosis in the wives of neurotic men. Part 1: symptomatology and personality. *British Journal of Psychiatry*, **122**, 33–43.

Ovenstone I.M.K. (1973b). The development of neurosis in the wives of neurotic men. Part 2: Marital role functions and marital tension. *British Journal of Psychiatry*, **122**, 711–717.

Parker G., Johnston P., Hayward L. (1988). Parental 'Expressed Emotion' as a predictor of schizophrenic relapse. *Archives of General Psychiatry*, **45**, 806–813.

Pattison E.M., De Francisco D., Wood P. et al. (1975). Psychosocial kinship model for family therapy. *American Journal of Psychiatry*, **132**, 1246–1251.

Perlman B., Hartman E.A. (1982). Burnout: Summary and future research. *Human Relations*, **35**, 283–305.

Platt S. (1985). Measuring the burden of psychiatric illness on the family: an evaluation of some rating scales. *Psychological Medicine*, **15**, 383–394.

Royal College of Psychiatrists (1980). Psychiatric rehabilitation in the 1980's. Report of the Working Party on Rehabilitation of the Social and Community Psychiatry Section.

Royal College of Psychiatrists. (1987). Psychiatric rehabilitation updated. *Bull. R.C. Psychiat.*, **11**, 71.

Rutter M.L., Brown G.W. (1966). The reliability and validity of measures of family life and relationships in families containing a psychiatric patient. *Social Psychiatry*, **1**, 38–53.

Salokangas R.K.R. (1983). Prognostic implications of the sex of schizophrenic patients. *British Journal of Psychiatry*, **142**, 145–151.

Scheff T.J. (1966). *Being Mentally Ill*. Chicago: Aldine.

Shakow D. (1973). Some thoughts about schizophrenic research in the context of high risk studies. *Psychiatry*, **36**, 353–365.

Shepherd G. (1984). *Institutional Care and Rehabilitation*. Longman Applied Psychology.

Shepherd G. (1986). Social skills training and schizophrenia. In *Handbook of Social Skills Training*, Vol. 2. (Hollin C.R., Trower P. eds.). London: Pergamon Press.

Shepherd G. (1988). The contributions of psychological interventions to the treatment and management of schizophrenia. In *Schizophrenia: the Major Issues*. (Bebbington P.E., McGuffin P. eds.). Oxford: Heinemann.

Smith J., Birchwood M.J. (1987). Specific and nonspecific effects of educational intervention with families living with a schizophrenic relative. *British Journal of Psychiatry*, **150**, 645–652.

Spivak G., Platt J., Shire M. (1976). *The Problem Solving Approach to Adjustment*. Washington DC: Jossey Bass.

Stevens B. (1972). Dependence of schizophrenic patients on elderly relatives. *Psychological Medicine*, **2**, 17–32.

Stevens B.C. (1973). Evaluation of rehabilitation for psychotic patients in the community. *Acta Psychiatrica Scandinavica*, **46**, 136–140.

Strachan A.M. (1986). Family intervention for the rehabilitation of schizophrenia. *Schizophrenia Bulletin*, **12**, 678–698.

Strachan A.M., Leff J.P., Goldstein M.J. et al. (1986). Emotional attitudes and direct communication in the families of schizophrenics: A cross-national replication. *British Journal of Psychiatry*, **149**, 279–287.

Strachan A.M., Feingold D., Goldstein M.J. et al. (1989). Is Expressed Emotion an index of a transactional process II. Patient's coping style. *Family Process*, **28**, 169–181.

Strang J.S., Falloon I.R.H., Moss H.B. et al. (1981). The effects of family therapy on treatment compliance in schizophrenia. *Psychopharmacology Bulletin*. **17**, 87–88.

Stricker K., Rook A., Buchkremer G. (1989). Expressed Emotion and course of disease in schizophrenic outpatients: Results of a two year follow-up in a German study. Paper presented at the 19th Annual Congress of the European Association of Behaviour Therapy, Vienna, Sept 20–24.

Sturgeon D., Turpin D., Kuipers L. et al. (1984). Psychophysiological responses of schizophrenic patients to high and low Expressed Emotion relatives: a follow-up study. *British Journal of Psychiatry*, **145**, 62–69.

Szmukler G.I., Berkowitz R., Eisler I. et al. (1987). Expressed Emotion in individual and family settings: a comparative study. *British Journal of Psychiatry*, **151**, 174–178.

Tarrier N., Vaughn C.E., Lader M.H. et al. (1979). Bodily reactions to people and events in schizophrenics. *Archives of General Psychiatry*, **36**, 311–315.

Tarrier N., Barrowclough C. (1987). A longitudinal psychophysiological assessment of a schizophrenic patient in relation to the Expressed Emotion of his relatives. *Behavioural Psychotherapy*, **15**, 45–57.

Tarrier N., Barrowclough C., Porceddu K. et al. (1988a). The assessment of psychophysiological reactivity to the Expressed Emotion of the relatives of schizophrenic patients. *British Journal of Psychiatry* **152**, 618–624.

Tarrier N., Barrowclough C., Vaughn C. et al. (1988b). The community management of schizophrenia: a controlled trial of a behavioural intervention with families to reduce relapse. *British Journal of Psychiatry*, **153**, 532–542.

Tennant C., Bebbington P.E., Hurry J. (1981). The role of life events in depressive illness: is there a substantial causal relation? *Psychological Medicine*, **11**, 379–389.

Tidmarsh D., Wood S. (1972). Psychiatric aspects of destitution. In *Evaluating a Community Psychiatric Service*, (Wing J.K., Hailey A.M. eds.). Oxford: Oxford University Press.

Tomaros V., Vlachonikolis I.G., Stefanis C.N. et al. (1988). The effect of individual psychosocial treatment on the family atmosphere of schizophrenic patients. *Social Psychiatry*, **23**, 256–261.

Tuckett D. (1982). Final report on the patient project. Health Education Council.

Turpin G., Tarrier N., Sturgeon D. (1988). Social psychophysiology and the study of biopsychosocial models of schizophrenia. In *Social Psychophysiology: Theory and Clinical Applications*, (Wagner H. ed.). Chichester: Wiley.

Valone K., Goldstein M.G., Morton J.P. (1984). Parental Expressed Emotion and psychophysiological reactivity in an adolescent sample at risk for schizophrenic spectrum disorders. *Journal of Abnormal Psychology*, **93**, 448–457.

Vaughn C.E. (1977). Patterns of interactions in families of schizophrenics. In *Schizophrenia: The Other Side*. (Katschnig H. ed.). Vienna: Urban and Schwarzenberg.

Vaughn C. (1986). Patterns of emotional response in the families of schizophrenic patients. In *Treatment of Schizophrenia: Family Assessment and Intervention*. (Goldstein M.J., Hand I., Hahlweg K. eds.). Berlin: Springer.

Vaughn C.E. (1989). Annotation: Expressed Emotion in family relationships. *Journal of Child Psychology*, **30**, 13–22.

Vaughn C., Leff J.P. (1976a). The influence of family and social factors on the course of psychiatric illness: a comparison of schizophrenic and depressed neurotic patients. *British Journal of Psychiatry*, **129**, 125–137.

Vaughn C.E., Leff J.P. (1976b). The measurement of Expressed Emotion in the families of psychiatric patients. *British Journal of Clinical and Social Psychology*, **15**, 157–165.

Vaughn C.E., Snyder K.S., Jones S. et al. (1984). Family factors in schizophrenic relapse: Replication in California of British research in Expressed Emotion. *Archives of General Psychiatry*, **41**, 1169–1177.

Venables P. (1977). Psychophysiological high risk strategy with Mauritian children: Methodological issues. Paper read at the Psychophysiological Conference, London.

Wallace C.J., Liberman R.P. (1985). Social skills training for patients with schizophrenia: a controlled clinical trial. *Psychiatry Research*, **15**, 239–247.

Waters M.A., Northover J. (1965). Rehabilitated long-stay schizophrenics in the community. *British Journal of Psychiatry*, **111**, 258–267.

Watts F.N., Bennett D.H. (1983a). *Theory and Practice of Psychiatric Rehabilitation*. Chichester. Wiley.

Watts F.N., Bennett D.H. (1983b). Management of the staff team. In *Theory and Practice of Psychiatric Rehabilitation* (Watts F.N., Bennett D.H. eds.), 313–328. Chichester: Wiley.

Watts S. (1988). A descriptive investigation of the incidence of high EE in Staff working with schizophrenic patients in a hospital setting. Unpublished dissertation. Diploma in Clinical Psychology, British Psychological Society.

Wig N.N., Menon D.K., Bedi H. et al. (1987a). The cross-cultural transfer of ratings of relatives' Expressed Emotion. *British Journal of Psychiatry*, **151**, 156–160.

Wig N.N., Menon D.K., Bedi H., et al. (1987b). The distribution of Expressed Emotion components among relatives of schizophrenic patients in Aarhus and Chandigarh. *British Journal of Psychiatry*, **151**, 160–165.

Wing J.K. (1982). Course and Prognosis of Schizophrenia. In *Handbook of Psychiatry. Vol. 3. Psychoses of Uncertain Aetiology*. (Wind J.K., Wing L. eds.). Cambridge: Cambridge University Press.

Wing J.K. (1987). Psychosocial factors affecting the long term course of schizophrenia. In *Psychosocial Treatment of Schizophrenia*, (Strauss J., Böker W., Brenner H. eds.). Stuttgart: Hans Huber.

Wing J.K. (1989). The concept of negative symptoms. *British Journal of Psychiatry*, **155**, (Suppl. 7), 10–14.

Wing J.K., Freudenberg R.K. (1961). The response of severely ill chronic schizophrenic patients to social stimulation. *American Journal of Psychiatry*, **118**, 311–322.

Wing J.K., Bennett D.H., Denham J. (1964a). *The Industrial Rehabilitation of Long Stay Schizophrenic Patients*, Medical Research Council Memo No. 42, London, HMSO.

Wing J.K., Monck E., Brown G.W. et al. (1964b). Morbidity in the community of schizophrenic patients discharged from London mental hospitals in 1959. *British Journal of Psychiatry*, **110**, 10–21.

Wing J.K., Brown G.W. (1970) *Institutionalism and Schizophrenia*, Cambridge: Cambridge University Press.

Wing J.K., Morris B., eds. (1981). *Handbook of Psychiatric Rehabilitation Practice*. Oxford: O.U.P.

World Health Organisation (1979). *Schizophrenia: An International Follow-up Study*. Chichester: John Wiley and Sons.

Wynne L.C., Singer M. (1963). Thought disorder and family relations of schizophrenics. *I. Archives of General Psychiatry*, **9**, 191–206.

Wynne L.C., Singer M. (1965). Thought disorder and family relations of schizophrenics. *II. Archives of General Psychiatry*, **12**, 187–212.

Yalom I.D. (1975). *The Theory and Practice of Group Psychotherapy*. New York: Basic Books.

Yarrow M., Clausen J., Robbins P. (1955a). The social meaning of mental illness. *Journal of Social Issues*, **11**, 33–48.

Yarrow M., Schwartz C.G., Murphy H.S. et al. (1955b). The psychological meaning of mental illness in the family. *Journal of Social Issues*, **11**, 12–24.

Zubin J., Magaziner J., Steinhauer J.R. (1983). The metamorphosis of schizophrenia: From chronicity to vulnerability. *Psychological Medicine*, **13**, 551–571.

Index